Swords and Saints

A Doctor's Journey

Robert Adams, MD

Published by Heroes Media Group

Printed in the United States of America

Book Design by Shannon Whittington
Cover Design by Thomas McPherson

Editorial assistance by Marie Hagen, Tom Clemmer, friends and patients.

ISBN
978-0-578-65488-1 (Paperback)
978-0-578-65488-8 (eBook)

1. Biography & Autobiography, Medicine, Military

About the Cover

The Navy Officer's sword traveled with me since I was a teenager at the U.S. Naval Academy. It represents duty, honor, strength, leadership, war, and love of country. My military experiences taught me lethal skills and discipline, which helped when I traded in the sword for a scalpel.

As a full-service Family Medicine doctor my scalpel and I participated in lots of surgeries and delivered hundreds of babies.

The white coat and stethoscope are symbols of a rewarding life in medicine. I wore them with my Army uniform, surgical scrubs, and later as a Knightdale, NC community physician with pride and great joy.

Blue is the color of the sea and sky where I worked and played during my military service and it symbolizes loyalty, truth, faith, and heaven.

The journey I share here has been diverse, exciting, and rewarding.

OTHER BOOKS BY ROBERT ADAMS

Six Days of Impossible Navy SEAL Hell Week a Doctor Looks Back
www.sealhellweek.com
Book 1 in *The Doctor* series.
Also available on Audible Audiobooks

Contents

> *"Out of the night that covers me*
> *Black as the pit from pole to pole,*
> *I thank whatever gods may be*
> *For my unconquerable soul."*
> *Invictus — William Henley*

Prologue

Doctor scrubs, a starched white coat, and a black stethoscope are all parts of a physician's uniform. I love uniforms. Any uniform will do - Cub Scouts at 8, Boy Scouts at 11, Eagle Scout at 14, Explorer Scout at 16, U.S. Naval Academy Midshipman at 17, Naval officer, then Army officer. Uniforms worn with pride make you stand straighter and walk with purpose.

From the Naval Academy until medical school I wore a Navy uniform.

I wore Army uniforms proudly for eighteen more years, added numerous medals and badges, and retired as a Medical Corps Colonel (O-6). The Army dress uniform, with all its shiny pieces, parts, bangles, and beads is still fun to wear.

Uniforms with awards, badges, medals, and sashes display personal accomplishments. Boy Scout awards like the one-mile swim, 50-mile hike, Order of the Arrow, God and Country, and Eagle Scout are saved and honored. Mine remind me of successes that I wanted and needed.

The military gave me jump wings (static line, freefall, and Korean jump wings), a Scuba Diver silver badge, Flight Surgeon silver wings, and a Navy SEAL big gold Eagle insignia. These acknowledged challenges taken and met. Others envied them. I loved them.

Boy scouts, summer camps, and sports gave me refuge away from a dysfunctional home life. I entered the U.S. Naval Academy at age seventeen. Lacrosse and wrestling had been my high school sports. Swimming was a hobby, and the Academy offered all this and more, so I tried to fit in but failed.

A desire for independence and control made me a square peg in a round hole. I would graduate anyway and later discover that these past obstacles overcome would serve me well. Hell Week in my SEAL training was six days of no sleep, soaking wet, freezing cold endurance that lead to extreme mental and physical exhaustion. It was hard, but not worse than I had experienced before.

The Navy years were rewarding - great times with amazing men. Parachuting, scuba diving, demolitions, weapons training, and endurance athletics made it exciting, but it was a young man's profession. I went to medical school at age thirty-six to keep that excitement alive.

My adventures as a civilian physician began after thirty-six years in a military uniform -- at age fifty-five.

One question that intrigued my family and friends was, "why did you walk this difficult and expensive path to a second career in medicine?"

It was due to a search for meaning. I wanted the same sense of fulfillment and excitement that I had enjoyed as a SEAL platoon commander. Medicine was never a calling, but it was, in retrospect, a destiny.

The following personal experiences helped me grow as a person and a physician. They involve patients that trusted me, and for that I will be forever grateful. Some make me laugh. Some make me cry or say *wow*.

They should not die with me.

Chapter 1 – Primum Non Nocere

Primum non nocere has always been my medical mantra. Hippocrates is credited with this dictum, and it means *First, do no harm.*

As I reflect on three decades as a doctor, I am reminded of how much fun I have had and am grateful to have studied and practiced medicine later in life.

Starting in my late thirties allowed me to benefit from past experiences. Younger students do four years of college, four years of medical school, and graduate into residency programs of three to seven more years to learn their specialty. They emerge from their all-consuming educational cocoons with limited life experience.

These years of learning are physically and financially exhausting, stressful, and isolated. There are few chances to experience the birth of a child, death of a loved one, or a job you hate. Patients will present for help with all these issues. Younger physicians are less than fully prepared.

Education does not help a physician understand loneliness, alcoholism, child abuse, bad bosses, financial crisis, addiction, or poverty.

In the age of the internet, there is a vast amount of information for those able to access it. An inquisitive person can often figure out what is wrong with themselves before seeking a doctor's advice and confirmation.

"Doctor" is a title that establishes credibility with persons in need or distress. That credibility comes with heavy responsibility as disease and psychiatric illnesses are everywhere. Airplanes bring infections. Water and food carry and spread germs, and alcohol, smoking, and sugar cause severe illnesses. Young and old often die too soon. After decades of learning from my patients, I have become a teacher. Doctors, physician assistants (PA) and nurse practitioners (NP) come for advice.

"Do I cut the abscess? Does she need to be in the hospital? Is this EKG showing ischemia? What should I do? Will this medication cause harm?" I have the experience to change lives. To ignore my advice can be harmful – a sin against the institution of healing.

Most physicians are quite good at what they do, but success is limited by what they know, and especially by what they don't know. Knowledge grows with experience, and without constant striving to keep current, a physician's knowledge becomes outdated. Technology bypasses some. Medical advances blow past what they were taught.

There is an increasing number of physician extenders providing medical care. These physician assistants and nurse practitioners provide needed access in a world with a growing population and not enough doctors.

I regularly encountered misdiagnoses, unnecessary tests, misuse of drugs, or other problems caused by well-intentioned but under-trained medical providers. Urgent care clinics are popping up manned only by physician extenders. A supervising physician might have oversight responsibility for forty to fifty extenders. Some states do not even limit the number of supervised physician extenders. It is a system doomed to failure.

Our health care insurance plans are inefficient and unfair. Insurance companies force providers to use medicines based on price and not on effectiveness. A better way is required - and inevitable.

I have observed doctors practicing in Iraq (the cradle of civilization), and other countries. In 2003, I met Iraqi doctors who had taken advantage of their country's free six-year medical education taught in English. The British had instituted this program in the 1920s after World War I.

Following medical school and an intern year, doctors in Iraq would serve twelve years as a general medical practitioner in outlying areas. They could return to a residency program and learn a specialty after serving and were paid about $100 a month for those first twelve years. There were no nurses or physician extenders.

They lived with their parents or in small clinics far from bigger cities with limited access to medications or specialists. When the U.S. brought more freedom to Iraq, there had been zero access to outside education for the previous twenty-five years. Saddam Hussein had made it illegal for doctors to leave the country as they often never returned. The Internet was forbidden, and libraries had few books.

These doctors learned at the bedside - the honored Hippocratic method. Teachers passed on what they could from memory or notebooks they carried. Iraq had once been the shining star in the Middle East medical world. But, after years of suppression, they practiced the way they had years before.

"Why do you do this?" I inquired of the doctors.

The answer was almost always the same. "I want to help my people."

I realized that these physicians were much like our American frontier doctors. In the early 1900s, U.S. doctors did everything. They were obstetricians and surgeons and family doctors. They were paid with pennies and chickens. They did it because they wanted to help others. They were honored and respected and often did their work for free. It was a calling in the highest sense of the word.

Technology continues to make each day more exciting and productive. It also makes it more dangerous. There are more treatment and testing options, and we can do so much more.

But there is much we should *not* do – just because we can. Pray that physicians continue to seek the wisdom to know the difference.

Primum non nocere.

Chapter 2 – Such Trust

"Knife to Doctor Adams," ordered the attending physician.

I reached out my scrubbed, sterile-glove-covered hand towards the surgical assistant. She slapped a shiny steel scalpel expertly onto my palm, and the sterile blade flashed in the bright lights. A soft rubber *plop* was all we heard. It was my moment. I would cut a deep, smile-shaped incision into the bulging abdomen of a living person.

I would dissect and manually tear through the muscles and layers of tissue to the uterus and open that now much-enlarged organ with another smaller incision. Out of the bleeding set of wounds would emerge a slippery baby covered with a film of whitish grease. I would lift a squirming child out of the warm wet hole, cut the cord, and announce, *It's a boy.* A new life would begin today.

As the nurse slapped my palm with the tools of our trade, she watched my hands for a tremor and my eyes for fear. She knew this was my first time as the primary surgeon. What she saw was steady hands and a look of awe. But I was shaking inside.

How have I earned her trust? I wondered, glancing over my paper mask to the anxious face of the now pain-free woman. The epidural anesthesia drip in her back left her numb from the waist down. In addition, the anesthesiologist was adding a steady flow of anti-anxiety medicine to her IV fluids. She was aware, chemically calm, and watching.

"We are going to start now," I announced while looking directly at her shiny blue eyes. Mine were bright blue also and concentrating.

Do she and her husband know how humbled I am by their belief in my newly developing skills? If they could hear my thoughts now, I wondered, would they tell me to stop? I was pretty sure they would.

A sterile blue-paper drape was placed neatly over her tummy. The drape had a peel-away piece of waxed paper protecting the clear adhesive window over her abdomen. The waxed paper was removed as we unfolded the drape into place and handed the upper edge of the blue paper to the anesthesiologist. He attached it to two poles at the head of the bed, creating a sterile barrier. He and the dad could stand behind it and listen. The surgical area was not visible. Watching could be most disturbing.

I placed the scalpel at the left lower edge of a plastic-covered pumpkin-sized bulge at a planned ninety-degree angle. My hand pressed down until I could see and feel the outer skin layers separate. The skin was brown from the pre-surgical Betadine paint job.

The temperature-controlled, frosty room reeked of disinfectant. Bright lights glared above and with one single deliberate movement I cut deeply and accurately along the path I had mapped in my head. The result was a bright red, curved incision, stretching ten inches along the bottom of the brown Betadine-stained abdomen. Dark red bubbles of blood oozed up along the incision, and the thick liquid turned shiny and more brightly red as it mixed with the oxygen in the air. The operating room technician dabbed at the incision.

"Nice job, Doctor," observed the tech with amazement in her voice.

The wide-eyed husband peeked over the paper drape. He could not see the procedure underway, and his eyes, peeking over his paper mask, showed confusion and expectation of his son's imminent arrival. I remembered how I had experienced the births of my two children, long before going to medical school. I had been confused and lost.

I wanted to reassure him, but it was not *my* operating room. It belonged to my mentor, and she concentrated on me. Four people were watching, and we all wore looks of alert concentration.

My decision to go to medical school had come late at thirty years old when my son was only two months old. My hair had been thinning since college, and there were strands of gray. A daughter was in our future when I came home and asked my wife Jeri for permission to go to medical school. I wanted adventure again and a greater sense of fulfillment.

I worked full time after finishing my MBA degree (no badge or button earned) and had gone to work for the corporate world. This was a place without morals or excitement where making money was the only objective. Weekends were spent doing Navy Reserves training, but this was not enough to meet my need for a sense of fulfillment.

"If we decide to do this, it will take a couple of years to get accepted. I'll have to go back to school at night after work, and if I get in, we'll have to sell everything and borrow money. We'll be poor for seven years of medical school and residency," I observed, with hope and reservation.

She was five foot four inches tall, intelligent, blond, and beautiful - the woman of my dreams. Her love for children and animals was why I needed her as my wife because I knew our children would be raised with compassion. She was feeding our son a bottle as she contemplated a response.

She knew I was not happy in my current job, where making money was my only task. Money has no ethics. To make one dollar, I had to get someone else to give it to me. When I commanded elite warriors parachuting, diving, shooting, and blowing things up in defense of our country, there was seldom a bad day. I would go to bed at night, distressed that I had to sleep eight hours before I could wake up and do it all again. I wanted to feel good again...like that.

"Sweetie, we were poor and happy when we got married, and we can be poor and happy again. I want you to come home and hug our kids. Anything less is unacceptable. You should try," she said with encouragement in her sparkling blue eyes.

"Besides, you probably won't get in at your age," she added with a bright smile, shifting our infant son to her other arm. She stood up straight, with a swimmer's shoulders and an athletic build. Her smile could light up any room. "Go for it anyway." Unbeknownst to either of us, our daughter was just beginning to flutter in her mommy's tummy.

Three and a half years later, I arrived at the Bowman Gray School of Medicine, Wake Forest University, in Winston-Salem, North Carolina, with a wife, two children, and everything we owned in our car and a small moving van. I was thirty-six years old.

But, this day, in the operating room, I gently lifted a newborn upward for all to see.

"It's a boy!" I announced proudly, and my voice cracked a bit.

Until the 1900s, Cesarean section deliveries were reserved as a last-ditch effort to save a baby when the mother died or was dying from childbirth. Mothers did not survive in part due to a belief that the physician should leave the uterus open *"to drain the evil humors."* Physicians believed that sutures would cause infections and that the uterus would contract back to normal and close by itself. This erroneous belief led to universal abdominal infection, sepsis, and death.

In the 1870s, surprisingly in the United States, a report came from frontier doctors that they had been sewing up the uterus with silver wire after C-section deliveries, and their patients had lived.

Their logic was reasonable. "Since the mother will certainly die, why not sew up the incision and see what happens?" they reasoned. It was scoffed at and ignored by medical teaching centers. Almost ten years later, these institutions of learning repeated the experiment to prove that the paper sent to them by these frontier doctors was wrong. The women lived.

Anesthesia using ether came along in 1846 but was seldom used in childbirth. Midwives sometimes quoted the Bible (Genesis 3:16) as requiring women to suffer in childbirth to atone for Eve's sin.

This false biblical prohibition lessened when Queen Victoria used chloroform for the births of her two children in 1853 and 1857.

Thank God.

"As a medical doctor, I have known the face of adversity. I have seen death and dying, suffering, and sorrow. I also remember the plight of students overwhelmed by their studies."
Russell M. Nelson

GETTING THERE

Chapter 3 - Dad, and Dying

I held my dad's hand as he died. His passing was peaceful, and, except for my mother, who held the other hand and kept sobbing the words *I love you*, it was quiet.

The breathing machine kept inflating his lungs, and it was difficult to believe he was dead, but the cardiac monitor above the bed had registered his last heartbeat. I had watched the peaks get farther apart until they stopped. It was then that I answered my mom, who was asking when we would know that he was gone.

"We know now, Mom. His heart has stopped."

He was only sixty-three years old, and he never knew I later went to medical school.

Dad was admitted to the hospital four days before his death for 'low back pain.' He had been in pain for months, but as far as we knew, he never sought a doctor's help. They had diagnosed his lung cancer some time before, but he did not tell us. It was terminal at the time of diagnosis. They planned nothing medical, except regular check-ups.

He had lived a hard life. He smoked a lot and drank even more. He flew fighters for the Navy and was a test pilot in his heart even after he flew a desk. He gave up alcohol with the help of Alcoholics Anonymous twelve years before he died, and he often left the house to meet with someone who called for help with drinking.

The strange thing about his last year was his response to our concern when we would see him grimace in pain. He would refuse to see a doctor.

"I'll let you know when it's time to go," he would reply.

We all knew something was wrong, and he knew too.

One day he was unable to move. "It's time to go," he stated.

During his first day in the hospital, he instructed me about his estate papers and told me where to find his insurance and official documents. It seemed silly. The doctors disclosed very little, and an autopsy was against Dad's wishes.

The last few days with my father were a mixture of surprise and amazement. He would awaken from vivid dreams about flying and tell me about them. Present-day astronauts had been his wingmen in squadrons past. He was reliving his best adventures with them. The peace on his face, as he told of the dreams, was confused by my presence at an older age. In his mind, I should have been younger or somewhere else.

They moved him to intensive care, and he fought to stay alive so the family could say goodbye. It was a real battle, and one evening his heart stopped.

"Don't do again – hurt!" read his note, after shocking him back to life.

"Please let me go. It's OK," he scribbled. He was intubated and could not speak.

We all admitted that the end was near.

Unobserved, I baptized him. I laid my hand on his head and made him welcome in heaven. He had never been a religious man, but I discovered later that he had learned to pray.

I kissed him. I did that for me as we had never kissed. I had wanted to kiss and hug him, but that task, for his three children, was delegated to our mom. Dad died as he had lived – strong and without emotion.

As his heart slowed, his eyes rolled back, and we closed his eyelids. His hands were cold, and the monitor recorded the last heartbeat. A full minute passed as I fought back the tears.

His eyes opened, pupils contracted, and he looked over at my mom.

I watched their eyes meet and hold for what seemed like an eternity but was only a few seconds. Then they closed again. It was clear to my mom what had happened. He had made one last monumental effort to say, "I hear you, and I love you too. Goodbye."

He taught me much as a child, but he taught me more with his passing. I suddenly knew that death was an inevitable part of life. It was not necessarily difficult or painful to die, and an overwhelming peace follows monumental suffering.

These lessons help me now with patient care and family coping issues. They give me a better perspective on life. I learned that death was in the future for all, and it helped distinguish the important from the trivial.

I saw the power of the mind in Dad's farewell glance. I learned, with certainty, that there was a soul. It lived on, somewhere outside the body left behind.

Thanks, Dad, for these final lessons that you never intended to teach me. *And guess what? I'm a doctor now. You'd be proud.*

The North Carolina Medical Journal published this chapter when I was a medical student. It was the winning student essay that year.

Chapter 4 - The Decision

Our family moved every three years during my formative years. We were in Yokosuka, Japan, when President Kennedy was shot and killed. It was a Boy Scout Jamboree day. Our troop produced a display on first aid, and I staffed the booth.

My uniform was ironed and creased, and my merit badge sash had fifteen neatly aligned badges of various colors and designs. My pocket rank patch was for First Class scout, with an eagle, an American flag shield, and two stars. At the bottom, it read, 'Be Prepared.'

"What do you do when someone has a seizure and is biting his tongue?" probed a wandering scout.

"You take your belt off and put it between his teeth," I responded, thinking instinctively.

"Oh. That would work," he responded, impressed. It surprised me I came up with an answer. It was not in my first aid book.

I made Eagle Scout at age fourteen. I loved scouting, as it got me out of a dysfunctional household and gave me a sense of accomplishment. When I had done all I could as a Boy Scout, I formed an Explorer Post. *Keep the fun alive* was my mantra then. I was curious about medical stuff, so I asked the military hospital in Pensacola, Florida, to sponsor our troop.

We had access to the inner workings of hospital-based medical care.

Then we moved again.

The family went to Belgium, and I went to a boarding school in Maryland. It was 1967, and I had decided to become a SEAL. Reader's Digest had published an article announcing the existence of this previously unknown secret organization. "Supercommandos of the Wetlands" had struck me straight in the heart.

I would be a frogman. If joining the Navy was necessary to do that, then following in our family's footsteps made sense. I would go to the Naval Academy, like Dad and Granddad.

At the Naval Academy, my grades were average. Graduation, not academic excellence, was the goal, but one class captured my imagination. I earned a 4.0 grade in biology and loved it. My professor enjoyed staying after class to help me revel in it more. This extra effort would factor into future life decisions.

I did not get one of the three slots for SEAL training offered to our class on Service Selection Night. Selection opportunities were based on class rank, and I was not high enough. The three available slots were gone when my number came up. I would need to drive a destroyer first. An older World War II-era destroyer, USS Hamner (DD-718), in San Francisco, awaited me. Launched in November 1945, she hid lots of ancient rust under her layers of grey paint.

I had thirty days of paid vacation to use before reporting, so I joined twelve classmates in Key West, Florida, for Underwater Swimmers School. We would all become Navy Scuba Divers. One of our instructors was a SEAL.

"Sir, you're having too much fun here. Have you ever thought of becoming a Navy SEAL?" he queried.

I smiled at the question.

Eighteen months later, in 1974, I began Basic Underwater Demolition/SEAL school. I graduated as one of eleven men out of the seventy that started and was the senior officer remaining.

In 1978, the post-Vietnam war period, the military shrank, and funding evaporated. I explored other options and transferred to the Reserve Teams, so I could get an MBA and try my hand at business.

I met the love-of-my-life in her hometown of Harrisonburg, Virginia, while starting my first business and going to school at James Madison University.

Three years later, we were married and moved to Washington, DC. I finished my degree and found a good job. We had a son eighteen months later.

Three years after our son's birth, I was accepted to medical school.

Let the good times roll! *Laissez les bon temps rouler.* Jeri and the two kids came along for the ride.

As we were driving to our new adventure, I asked my wife why she had married me, and I honestly wanted to know the answer. We were starting over again. I reminded her that I had barely a nickel to my name when I proposed.

Her answer tickles me to this day.

"I married you for your potential," she responded with a smile.

Chapter 5 – Childbirth

My first witnessed childbirth occurred long before I ever thought about medical school. It involved my wife and our son.

We had been married for two years. My wife was twenty-eight years old and pregnant, and we were doing all the right things. We exercised often, ate a proper diet, and drank no alcohol. We attended the hospital's recommended Lamaze classes. Our class had six couples, all due about the same time, and there were three classes left to participate in when Jeri phoned me.

"My water broke," she stated calmly.

"What are you talking about? You're not due yet!" I stammered.

It was 1 A.M. on Saturday, and I had just climbed into bed at the officer's quarters. I was scheduled for a weekend of Navy training, with our home now four hours away. The doctor had assured us that Jeri was not showing any signs of early labor risk.

We had an animated discussion that began with my disbelief and ended with her correcting my understanding of the situation.

"Sweetheart, trust me, the puddle of fluid at my feet right now could have no other cause. I'm not contracting much right now, so why don't you get a few hours of sleep and head back after the sun is up? I'll call you if labor starts for real," she stated, with a touch of excitement.

After a hurried phone call to my commanding officer, I slid back into bed and willed myself to sleep. There would be an adventure in the morning with four hours racing back home. My speed exceeded the posted limit as I rehearsed the story that I would tell the officer if I got stopped. I was unclear what would happen next, as we had not gotten that far in our Lamaze classes.

Contractions were in an irregular pattern, and her doctor said it was OK to wait until I got back to go to the labor deck if the contractions remained light and intermittent. *Labor deck* is the name for the maternity ward in a military hospital. Each previous doctor visit had included a urinalysis, a blood pressure check, and an ultrasound fetal heart rate measurement. The fetal heart rate usually stayed around 160, and the old wives' tale, quoted by the nurses, was that this meant we would have a girl. Boys had heart rates below 150, they suggested. The early week-thirteen ultrasound had not given us a sex determination, so we had a list of favorite girl names picked out.

I arrived back home at about 10:30 in the morning and found my lovely wife sound asleep.

"Honey, I'm home," I stated, in a slightly confused voice.

"Oh, hi," she responded sleepily. "I'm barely feeling the contractions. The doctor said we could wait until the afternoon to go to the labor deck for a checkup unless the contractions get strong and regular."

We both lay in bed with anticipation. Our daughter was coming today.

Four hours later, at the labor deck, we were advised to walk around for a while and see if the contractions got stronger. We walked all afternoon with little change. That evening we returned and were admitted for observation. If no fever or other problems developed, we could wait for nature to take its course. If twenty-four hours passed after the water broke, the doctor routinely helped nature along by adding medicine to make the contractions harder and faster. We were already past the twenty-four-hour mark since the water had broken, but we wanted a natural delivery.

The next morning our Lamaze class wandered by our room on their Sunday labor deck orientation.

"What are you doing here?" probed one of the ladies. "I'm due a week before you are."

We explained the situation, laughed with them, and waved as they moved on.

The doctor came by and announced it was time to start an IV drip to encourage stronger contractions. Jeri had a temperature of 100.4 degrees. He ordered antibiotics and suggested that they could begin an epidural pain management drip. We reminded him we were planning a more natural delivery for our first child, so they put the epidural on hold.

The contractions started getting harder and faster. The nurse would come in periodically, see Jeri doing her breathing and puffing, and ask again if she wanted an epidural for pain.

"No," we would both declare, but the resolve in her voice weakened a bit each time.

The nurse started checking the cervix for dilation. It needed to dilate to ten centimeters before she could start pushing. The pushing part could last up to two hours. She had dilated to five centimeters.

After another hour of contractions every three minutes – that lasted about thirty seconds each -- she leaned her head towards me and gave me an unmistakably pleading look.

"Nurse, we need drugs here!" I yelled out the door. She popped right in and smiled at us.

"Well, it's about time," she smiled. "I will get the anesthesiologist here right away." She left, and the look of relief on Jeri's red face was comforting.

The epidural took a few minutes to place. It worked fast, and the room got quieter. The contractions continued silently, and she stopped sweating. Her honey-blond hair remained pasted to her temples as she drifted off to sleep. She had dilated to seven centimeters.

It took three more hours before the nurse announced she was fully dilated and could start the pushing phase. The head of the bed was raised, and the nurse began coaching Jeri on how to push. It was difficult because she could not sense the contractions, or feel her muscles, to know if she was pushing or not. We had to watch the contraction monitor. When it showed a contraction starting, Jeri would try to help by simulating a bowel movement.

"Push!" the nurse and I would encourage when the monitor signaled a contraction. They were coming every three minutes, and she began sweating again with the effort.

"Stop pushing now," ordered the nurse firmly. She anxiously watched something on the monitor.

"Don't push, honey. I'm going to get the doctor to take a look." She disappeared and returned with the doctor in tow.

The white-coated doctor was smiling calmly as he examined the paper tracing produced by the monitor. He requested fresh sterile gloves and did his own check of the dilated cervix and found the baby's head.

"It appears we will have your baby soon, so we will move you to the delivery room." He turned to the nurse and said, "I may need to use forceps."

Everything happened fast. The bed rolled down the hall with me following. The nurse gave me a mask, gown, and paper booties to put on. The nurse already had hers in place.

The delivery room was cold, brightly lit, and smelled like antiseptic. The doctor moved to a stool placed at the foot of the bed. Jeri's feet dangled in cloth-covered metal stirrups, and her buttocks rested at the end of the bed table. Her knees remained bent to ninety degrees and leaned out away from her body, making room for the doctor to scoot in and work up close and personal.

The monitor showed the contractions and the baby's heart rate. When the contractions started, the baby's heart rate went down. This was different, and the doctor was not happy about it.

"I need to get your child out right now," he stated resolutely after watching another contraction with the same result.

"I am going to use forceps to grab the baby's head, and pull while you push," he instructed urgently.

"Nurse, I need you to push on her tummy, and help me get this baby out."

The nurse nodded, placed her two fists at the top of the bulging, baby-filled abdomen, and pushed down with all her might. Jeri turned her head towards me and puked out the yellow bilious contents of her stomach. The doctor pulled hard on his metal-handled forceps. Slowly a head emerged. A gush of fluid and blood followed.

"OK, stop pushing. The head is out, but there's some cord around its neck." He pulled out blue plastic clamps, placed them on the cord, cut between the clamps, and unwrapped the three loops of cord around our child's neck. The rest of our baby slipped slowly into his lap.

"It's a boy," he muttered automatically as he suctioned the mouth and nose with a blue rubber bulb. He handed the child to a waiting pediatric nurse who moved quickly to a table on wheels. She had been called to the delivery room as soon as we had arrived. My eyes widened in surprise. Jeri was busy throwing up.

Both nurses were working furiously at the pediatric table, and their arms were flailing all over the place.

I had expected to hear a cry. I was trying to digest the fact that we had a son and was confused.

"What's going on," I asked, in alarm. "Why isn't he crying?"

Our nurse paused, squinted over her shoulder at me, and said, "We are breathing for your baby right now."

I did not find that at all reassuring, and Jeri was dry heaving. This was not how I envisioned a delivery would happen.

I heard a cry. It was weak but audible.

Both nurses stopped what they were doing, grabbed the bassinet on wheels, and rushed it out of the room to the pediatric ICU where a neonatology doctor waited.

The obstetrician seated between my wife's legs focused on his sewing task. There was lots of blood on his hands and instruments. Nothing was happening like I thought it would, so I moved down the table to stand beside the doctor.

He glanced up at me, with instruments in both hands, and whispered, "Most daddies don't come down here."

I paused for a second and replied, "Well, this daddy is going to medical school soon, and honestly wants to know what's going on."

"Ah, in that case, sir, put on clean gloves, and hold this suture for me." The nurse appeared promptly with a pair of sterile gloves, and she helped me get them on. Size 7 ½. How she knew my glove size, I guessed, was from experience. I held the suture, and the doctor began a mini-lecture on fourth-degree vaginal tears and how to repair them. I was enthralled.

Our son came through the ordeal fine. There were issues related to the umbilical cord wrapped three times around his neck. His head was purple when it had emerged. There were bruises on both sides of his head from the forceps that had yanked him into the world. He would have to stay an extra few days under ultraviolet lights because of elevated bilirubin levels. The pediatrician had been concerned, but that resolved naturally.

He went home with us, discharged as "baby boy Adams," because we had never considered boy names, and could not agree on one with such short notice.

A few days later, we decided to follow family tradition, honor my father, and name him Robert Stark Adams, III. We agreed to call him "Trey."

Thirty-five years later, his son, Robert Stark Adams, IV would be born.

"The art of medicine consists of amusing the patient, while nature cures the disease."
Voltaire

WAKE FOREST UNIVERSITY MEDICAL SCHOOL

Chapter 6 – First Medical School Delivery

It took three years to go back to school at night and retake all the courses required for medical school admission. I worked a full day and went to classes at night. Chemistry, physics, biology, and biochemistry were already on my college transcript, but they were over ten years old, and that was not acceptable.

When researching how to get accepted, I learned I would need to retake all these classes. That was fine with me for two reasons. First, I would need coursework refreshed to pass and excel on the required MCAT (Medical College Admission Test). Second, my undergraduate grades were not good enough, so I made sure I got a 4.0 on all these repeated classes.

I applied to fourteen medical schools. Invitations to an interview came from only three.

My home state of Virginia came through for me in January. Medical College of Virginia said *yes*. It was in Richmond, Virginia, and located downtown in a rough neighborhood. Jeri was accepting, but not pleased with the location.

The same week I received a letter from Wake Forest University, Bowman Gray School of Medicine, stating that I had been put on a standby list.

I reacted quickly and fired off a request for a medical school scholarship to the Navy and the Army. That request could not be sent until the applicant was accepted to a school.

I sent my acceptance letter and fee to Richmond and waited anxiously for word from the armed services.

One month later, I had two offer letters. The Navy offered me a three-year scholarship, and the Army offered me four years.

With those letters in hand, I wrote to Wake Forest University. I had an unconventional plan.

"Dear sirs:

Please find enclosed a check for the required admission fee. I am on your standby list. I have been accepted to the Medical College of Virginia, but Wake Forest University is my first choice.

Please consider me for acceptance in your next class. I have received a full military scholarship and will not need any financial assistance.
Thank you for your kind consideration.
Sincerely,
Robert S. Adams, MBA"

My plan worked. The acceptance letter from the Bowman Gray School of Medicine arrived the next week. All medical schools were expensive, and Wake Forest was no exception. They liked the military scholarships because they freed up other scholarship money for the many students in need.

I restarted my military career by accepting a commission as an Army Second Lieutenant (O-1) to begin school as a medical student. This was a significant change since I wore the rank of Commander (O-5) in the Navy.

The Dean of Students was a Navy Rear Admiral, and I asked him to swear me in. He was pleased to do it. I showed up in my summer white Navy uniform, with Jeri and our two young children, Cori and Trey, ages two and a half and four-years old in tow.

When he completed swearing me in, he gazed at the family and me with curiosity. "Bob, I'm always pleased to welcome our students into the military. But I just turned a Navy SEAL Commander into an Army Second Lieutenant medical student. Honestly, I am having a hard time wanting to congratulate you," he smiled while shaking my hand.

Whether I had chosen Navy or Army, my rank would be reset to an O-1, per the terms of their scholarships. The military did not want or need new doctors graduating with prior higher ranks. Future assignments were rank dependent, and new doctors needed experience in entry-level jobs.

I did not like it, but I realized the necessity later.

School started in August for our class of 109. We were excited, first-year medical students. Eighteen of us volunteered to be in a new program Wake Forest University was developing. It allowed us to see, and do, clinical and medical activities, starting on the first month of school. The others were left with the lectures and long hours of memorization and study typical of the first two years of traditional medical school. But we were part of a new 'Parallel Curriculum' that allowed for supervised independent study and actual interaction with patients from day one. It was an experiment, and, as willing students, we were taking a chance that we would learn enough to pass our board exams at the end of the second year.

One month into our new adventure, Rick and I were standing behind a large glass window watching a Cesarean section baby delivery. The room was brightly lit, and we were watching two doctors, an anesthesiologist, and a dad, all dressed in gowns and masks.

We were fascinated with the show on display before us. The doctors were delivering a baby surgically. A baby emerged, in the hands of one of the surgeons, and the wide-eyed dad glowed. *This was awesome,* we thought while glancing around with glee to take it all in.

The show was far from over. The nurse wrapped her charge in blankets, while the doctors worked intently on their patient. A doctor reached back into the hole he had created and pulled out what appeared to be a blood-covered brown football. He placed it on the mother's stomach and began to sew on it.

Our eyes bulged, and I turned to Rick and asked, "What the heck is that?"

He thought, and guessed, "Do you suppose that is the uterus?"

We concluded that it was and continued to watch in amazement. We digested the fact that an organ that began as the size of a closed fist was now the size of a football. And that was after it had delivered its contents to the world.

"Wow," we both muttered.

Chapter 7 – Anatomy Lab

I snuck into the third-floor anatomy dissection room with my five-year-old son. The room reeked heavily of nose-burning formaldehyde. The lights were dim, and the partially dissected bodies lay in stainless-steel, covered containers. We were not supposed to be there, but it would not be the last rule I would break in training.

"OK, son, are you ready to see a dead body?" I whispered challengingly.

"Um, yes, I guess," he whispered. I had told him about my medical school classes, and this part caught his attention. He did not know what dissection meant, but he knew about death.

I lifted the heavy stainless top and revealed a grayish-brown shriveled corpse whose abdomen showed the surgical scars of exploration. The skin flaps had been returned to their normal anatomic positions.

"OK, I saw it. Thanks, Dad," he mumbled as he backed away. I closed the lid, sniffed at the unpleasant formaldehyde odor surrounding us, and tiptoed back to where we had come from.

"Don't tell mom," I suggested.

He probably would anyway, and I would be in trouble once again.

The next day found me back in the anatomy lab, ready to work on my assigned body. We had been instructed in the respect due to these donated remains. We took that seriously. The next many years ahead would be dedicated to learning how to prevent, or delay, the death we were witnessing today. The physicians that cared for our cadavers when they were alive had done all they could. Now they were ours to study.

I cut into the middle of the left lung in search of the main bronchial tube. I watched the liver-like, firm, grayish tissue part and reveal the tapered tube of the bronchial airway. What surprised me was the color of the lung tissue that folded out of the way. It was spotted black.

"He must have been a smoker," I commented to my lab partner. She nodded in agreement.

"Doctor Bo, can you tell from this black color that he was a smoker?" I asked.

Doctor Bo was a legend in the anatomy world. We often saw him puffing on his pipe while walking pensively outside. Today he ambled over knowingly and glanced at our dissection.

"That is a classic example of what a city dweller's lung can look like. The black is from carbon deposits, from all the soot and pollution found in the city air. A smoker's lung will be less solid, and often resemble a sponge, with holes visible throughout both lungs where the tobacco gasses have permanently dissolved the lung tissue," he instructed.

"That is the definition of emphysema," he continued. "God gave us two lungs when he added tobacco to the world. We can destroy one full lung's worth of functional capacity before we must go on oxygen. It's like we have a spare designed into the body system." He smiled and shuffled over to the next table.

It was a time for learning, and it was like drinking from a firehose. There was so much to absorb. The days and nights were filled with reading, lectures, note-taking, and discussions with professors and fellow students. There would be a national test at the end of our second year that must be passed to proceed on to our third year of school. The third year was when we would begin our clinical rotations in hospital and outpatient settings. Anatomy would be a big part of the test.

Anatomy lab was a formal class for both curriculums. Our group of eighteen met separately from the ninety others in our class for dissection and testing. Memorization of organs, vessels, bones, and nerves was required. It was exhausting and required long nights of study. My favorite study aid was an anatomy coloring book. I could color each page with colored pencils to visually separate the nerves, vessels, tendons, and muscles. It made a visual image that helped the memorization process.

Future surgeons in our class would return to dissect a knee or a hip. The resource was invaluable, and the sense of awe, when working on someone's donated body, never lessened.

Chapter 8 – Sutures and Pap Smears

"See one, do one, teach one," stated my mentor.

A four-week rotation in family medicine was built into our first-year curriculum, and the doctor I was assigned to shadow was sewing up a cut on his patient's leg. My job was to dab the wound and cut the black nylon sutures.

"Do you know that there are two ways to cut a suture? Any surgeon will tell you this. When you're in your surgery rotation, you will discover that as the assistant, you either cut the suture *too long or too short*." He smiled, and so did his patient. I snipped the suture.

"Perfect," said the doctor.

"Practice using instruments to tie knots, and you can do the next laceration we see."

I practiced on an orange. The next laceration came the following day. It was a farmer, and he had an inch-long cut at the base of his thumb. We could see the fat pad under the skin.

"OK, this is yours to sew," he said. He left the room, and I opened the suture kit.

I drew up Lidocaine into a 3-cc syringe and replaced the large 18-gauge needle with a smaller and shorter needle. My patient appeared relieved to see the smaller needle.

"OK, sir, I'm going to inject numbing medicine into your hand so we can close this cut up with a few stitches. Is that OK?"

"Sure, Doc."

I could see the skin around his cut turning white as the Lidocaine infused the skin. The drug had epinephrine in it to constrict blood vessels and make bleeding less. I had already learned from watching my mentor that white skin was also rapidly numb.

"All done. Did that hurt?" I asked.

"Just a little bee sting. No pain at all now."

I grabbed the stainless-steel needle driver tool, opened the 4-0 nylon suture pouch, and grabbed the middle of the curved needle as I had practiced. I touched his hand with the tip of the needle lightly.

"Do you feel anything where I'm touching?"

"Just a little pressure, Doc."

"Here we go," I said coolly while shaking a bit inside.

The needle slid neatly into the skin, under the incision and out the other side exactly where I wanted it to. The patient's face hovered over the table with his hand palm-up between us.

I took the needle driver off the back of the needle and grabbed the tip now protruding from the far side of his cut. *Piece of cake.*

I remembered that the first tie needed to be a 'surgeon's knot' with two loops of suture so the knot would not slip. I took the loose suture line and wrapped it expertly around the needle driver, then grabbed the free suture and pulled gently upwards. There was no knot. *Oops.*

"Let me do that again," I said, smiling and repeated the procedure as I remembered with the same result. No knot.

I don't know what I am doing wrong. He's watching me. What do I do now? Well, I know how to tie a shoe, and that results in the same kind of knot. I placed the needle driver down on the tray and grabbed the needle in one hand and the suture on the side closest to me in the other. Then I tied a simple knot and pulled it tight. The skin slid neatly together. I tied a couple more knots, grabbed the scissors and cut the suture precisely as I wanted it. One done, and two to go. *I can just do it this way for now.*

I grabbed the needle driver and loaded the needle again.

"How many of these have you done before today?" asked the more intent farmer. I smiled and changed the subject.

After I had tied all three sutures like a shoelace, it looked perfect. I put Bacitracin on it and wrapped it with sterile gauze. The doctor came back in, gave post-op care instructions, and asked him to come back in a week to have the sutures removed.

I pulled out another suture and tried to tie an instrument-assisted knot again. I did it slowly and watched myself carefully. It had worked on the orange yesterday. I realized that I had forgotten to release the driver from the needle. I was supposed to wrap the suture two times around the driver, and then let go of the needle. With the now free tip of the driver, I could grab the bitter end of the suture and pull it back through the two loops. *Voila.* A knot.

Now I was an expert and ready to teach a classmate how to do it. See one, do one, teach one.

The next morning's schedule was nothing but pap smears. Each patient we saw was advised that I was a student.

"My student will examine one breast and I will examine the other. I will recheck his exam," explained the doctor. The patients all nodded or mumbled their agreement. It was slightly uncomfortable for us all.

I followed the exam protocol as instructed. There was a nurse chaperone present to help with the pap smear that followed – all very professional and by-the-book.

As the morning progressed, I found myself watching my blank-faced mentor more intently. *Did he even notice that each room contained a half-naked woman? If this is what happens after a time in my chosen profession, maybe I need to rethink my plan?*

Lunchtime was approaching, and we were walking down the hallway. The doctor stopped, looked back at me and answered my unasked question, "I did notice."

Thank goodness. The rest of the day went by in a blur.

Over the years, I have diagnosed multiple cervical and breast cancers or infections. The undressed exams are sometimes embarrassing, but they are necessary and clinically relevant. The same is true of my female colleagues that search for and find enlarged prostates, hernias, rectal pathology, and testicular disease.

Chapter 9 - Two Years of Books

The first two years were jammed with essential studies and tests. The library became my home. Our unique program centered on meetings three times a week, where we would examine a patient scenario that always involved an illness. There were pictures and laboratory tests available, but a diagnosis was not.

With help from our physician mentors, we would break the case into areas of study, including anatomy, physiology, microbiology, biochemistry, and laboratory analyses. We would establish learning goals specific to the patient and his condition. It made the necessary study more realistic and relevant.

For the following two days after our planning session, we would study individually. We learned where all the best resource books were in the library. I would start early and often end late but could go home if I wanted to, for lunch or dinner, which made the process more tolerable. That was usually not so for our traditional curriculum classmates.

"I can't do this!" screamed and cried my study buddy, Lisa Miller. She lay flat on her back in her living room, sobbing and kicking her hands and feet. "It's impossible! How can we be expected to learn all this stuff?" she sniffled.

We had been trying to learn the minute details of cellular biology for the last four hours. The words were foreign. The amount of data was more than intimidating. The test was tomorrow for Lisa and the other regular curriculum students. Her dark hair was plastered to a sweaty forehead. Her eyes were red, and tears streaked her cheeks. Lisa was an invaluable friend who loved our children and felt like part of the family. Her poetry was always dark and haunting. It was her escape from the pressures of study. She would survive and thrive as a pediatrician in the town where she grew up, but that day we both wondered if graduation was even possible.

The Parallel Curriculum students did not take traditional tests. We were blessed to some extent, but we would need to know the same information to pass the United States Medical Licensing Exam (USMLE) Part 1. Failure of that national test would result in a release from medical school. Two expensive years would be gone and wasted if that happened.

We made every effort to learn and share learning. Designated note-takers in each lecture class shared notes with the rest of the class. Study groups met consistently to rehearse and share memorization tools.

"Scared Lovers Try Positions That They Can't Handle" was a mnemonic to help memorize the eight bones in the wrist: "Scaphoid, Lunate, Triquetrum, Pisiform, Trapezium, Trapezoid, Capitate, and Hamate."

Other mnemonics helped us memorize the twelve cranial nerves of the brain. We could examine each nerve for function during a physical exam. Sometimes our cases would mention a deficiency involving a cranial nerve. That would take us down a pathway of study that often led to diagnostic surprises.

"The patient has two different sized pupils," I noted. "That must be significant. A cranial nerve controls pupil size," I said to the study group. Our proctor watched.

"Brain tumor, chemical eye drops, eye infections, trauma, congenital disabilities, and surgery could all cause this. Do we know if it's a pre-existing condition?" solicited Linda. She was still a practicing Army Certified Registered Nurse Anesthetist (CRNA). She worked holidays and weekends in our hospital operating room to earn overtime money to help pay for medical school. We were the same age, thirty-six, but she had refused the military scholarship option. She held the rank of Lieutenant Colonel.

Linda was thin, athletic, and full of energy. She planned to be a trauma surgeon. After analyzing the data provided, we all focused on the color photo of a forty-four-year-old white male. His nose was large, and he had a ruddy complexion. Most engaging were his two pupils. They were not symmetric. That was likely one of our clues to the pending diagnosis.

"He could have syphilis," Linda continued. "It causes anisocoria and something called Adie's pupils. I've seen it before in the troops overseas when I deployed," she added matter-of-factly.

"Huh?" we responded. "Can you spell that?"
She had real-world experience and knowledge that few of us had. The proctor smiled in surprise.

"Linda, you can take a look at the lab information now since you nailed his diagnosis. The RPR or rapid plasma regain blood test, is positive. He has syphilis. Now let's make a list of the learning points, including treatment, and addressing his risk factors physically and psychologically," he directed.

We all began making notes and assigning responsibility. Some of us would research the illness, others the anatomy, physiology, behavioral health, and epidemiology. We were having fun learning about real medical conditions in a personal growth environment.

Down the hall were our ninety classmates stacked in raised, tiered rows of seats, making notes of the many items they would be required to memorize that day. This would continue for two grueling years.

"I passed the boards!" began my excited phone call home. The Part 1 USMLE results were in, and we had all passed. Both traditional and Parallel Curriculum students had made the cut.

"That's great, sweetheart. I guess that the study course you took paid off. The money was well spent, it seems."

I had taken a six-week course in my spare time doing practice test after practice test with a private agency that specialized in readying students for this critical exam.

The past two years had been challenging, and we had survived to progress to our third-year clinical phase.

"Darkness swallowed me
again today while the sun shone.
I hate it, but I let it win,
again and again
darkness wins.
I'm afraid one day I will not stand
back up again,
the war will be over and
darkness the victor." ~ Lisa Miller MS-1 (traditional
curriculum)

"The best doctors give the least medicines."
Benjamin Franklin

CLINICAL YEARS

Chapter 10 – HIV Blood Draw

Our third year began fast and furious, starting with an exciting and demanding week on the internal medicine wards. The pockets of the short white coat that marked me as a medical student bulged on both sides with books on drugs, laboratory guides, medicine and antibiotic treatment instructions, reflex hammer, penlight, and more. I wore it every day, and it collected viruses and bacteria alike. When I wore it home, I brought those germs with me. My children got sick more often as a result until I learned how to wash it. Resident physicians and attending physicians sported the classic longer white coat. Patients rarely recognized the difference.

Mornings started early before the resident in charge of our ward came in. We gathered labs, reviewed yesterday's orders and results, ran to radiology to look at X-rays, made notes on cards to introduce the patient at morning rounds, and consulted each other on what to do next. It was fun and exciting. What we needed to learn was monumental. What we studied each day built an expanding skill set that slowly made us appear knowledgeable and capable. Nothing could have been further from the truth.

Our team of students and residents gathered on the ward at 7 AM and moved from room to room. First, a student would present the current information on the patient.

I started. "Mr. Creech is a thirty-two-year-old white, HIV positive male admitted two days ago for fever and cough. His CD4 white blood cell count is very low, at 34. The X-ray is suspicious for pneumocystis pneumonia, but cultures are still pending."

I listed his meds and noted it was his fourth admission in the last five months. I added that his male friend was found in bed with him this morning, and the nurse told me they were having some kind of sex last night. No one seemed surprised, except me.

"Mr. Adams, please tell us about PCP and HIV, please," directed the resident. I responded with a quick summary of what I had read that morning about pneumocystis pneumonia.

"PCP is a fungal type infection, common in persons with impaired immune systems and a bad omen since natural immunity is needed to help in fighting any infection," I began. They all listened supportively.

We moved to the next room, and the next, until each of the three students had two or three patients to manage. The residents left us to do the blood draws, sputum cultures, nasogastric tube insertions, constipation manual stool disimpactions, catheter insertions and removals, and other needed activities to help the doctors and nurses care for our charges.

"Mr. Creech, I'm Bob Adams, your medical student. I need to draw blood for this morning's labs," I stated self-assured, as I put on a second pair of rubber gloves over the gloves I had on. The protocol required double gloves when drawing blood on HIV-infected patients.

I was nervous, and the patient watched me without comment. I pulled the brown rubber strap from my pocket, wrapped it above his elbow, cleaned the arm with alcohol swabs twice, laid a Band-Aid partially open on the bed, and pulled out the 10-cc syringe with an 18-gauge needle attached. I had a red top and a blue-top glass collection tube ready to transfer the blood into.

As I withdrew the needle from his arm, he saw an opportunity, and purposely moved his arm such that the needle slid into my thumb. I jerked back, looking wide-eyed to see if the needle had drawn blood. A red stain showed under the double layer of rubber gloves. I froze. The patient watched pleased.

It stunned and confused me. *What do I do now? He has AIDS,* I thought in shock. The only course of action I knew was to remove the gloves and wash the wound. I left the room and rushed to a sink at the nurse station, removed my gloves and washed vigorously with soap and water, found an alcohol pad nearby, and held the pad on my thumb with my index finger. I remembered that one training lecture had mentioned injecting the puncture site with Betadine. I found some Betadine, soaked a gauze pad and held it on my thumb. My heart beat fast, and my confusion increased.

I approached the nurse on duty and told her of my predicament. She was not surprised and told me I needed to report to the Infectious Diseases Department for care and reporting.

I knew where that office was, so I walked there with my thoughts spinning.

"You are needle stick number 109 this year," the secretary noted as she wrote in her logbook.

"What do I do now?" I whispered.

What followed was unscripted. I found an available doctor, and we discussed a plan. He would give me expensive HIV drugs saved from a patient that had died. I would take that until it ran out and check back for more. The Betadine injection was ruled out as too tissue destructive. I would need to use condoms for six months and get rechecked to determine if I had been infected with the AIDS virus. Medical students did not have insurance or workmen's compensation coverage. After noting there was nothing left to do, I returned to the ward.

I found the resident they assigned me to, told him where I had been, and he directed me to resume my duties. I had other patients to draw blood on. That was the student's job this morning, as the resident had more important things to do. I examined my list of patients and noticed that two more HIV-positive patients needed blood draws. The phlebotomist had taken care of Mr. Creech while I was gone.

I double gloved again, careful not to dislodge the betadine-soaked Band-Aid on my thumb, gathered my syringe, needle, alcohol pad, and red top tube and entered the next room. I explained I was a student there to draw blood and began my task. I placed the rubber band above the elbow, cleaned the antecubital space, and moved the needle forward.

My hand was shaking, and my mind fogged. I paused. After a moment of confusion and embarrassment, I removed the rubber band from his arm, excused myself, and went outside. I stood there, confused and scared for a few minutes thinking about the last few hours.

"Jim," I said to my resident. "I have not been trained on how to draw blood. This isn't the place for me to learn. I need to speak with someone in Administration about it."

He expressed sympathy and frustration, but he let me go. I had made his job a bit harder, but he would task the other students with doing what I would not.

It was time to do research. I went to the library, my favorite place of refuge, and found the medical center written guidelines for clinical operations and needle sticks. It was vague, but it stated that the medical center was responsible for the safety of clinical and training operations.

I had been a leader of men in the most demanding of environments, earned a master's degree in business, and needed to let someone know we had a problem.

Military training had taught me to start with the decision-maker. I walked slowly and deliberately to the hospital CEO's office. He was leaving as I arrived.

"Doctor Janeway, may I speak with you, please?" I began. He recognized me in my short white student's coat and surprised me by remembering my name.

"Of course, Bob. How can I help?" His childhood actor's smile was sincere and captivating.

I outlined the events of the day.

I expressed my concern about a lack of protocol for treating needle sticks. I then remarked with worry that I had been given no training on how to draw blood and asked if he had read the document about medical center responsibility I held in my hand. He had signed it.

"Of course, I have." He stated firmly, and with annoyance at my impertinence.

"I learned how to draw blood on the wards, and you students will too," he grumbled with authority thinking that would end the conversation. He leaned away.

"Sir, you did not have AIDS on your wards when you were a student. I will have to use condoms with my wife for the next six months until I find out if I have been infected. As a student, I'm not covered by workmen's compensation, and the hospital has no insurance that can cover the expensive drugs I need to take. They gave me a dead man's drugs."

That caused him to pause.

"Respectfully, Doctor Janeway, if I convert to HIV positive my career is over. I'm certain they will find the hospital liable, and although I might die, I expect I'll receive a large multimillion-dollar settlement. Multiply that times 109 students, and it would be cheaper to train us in phlebotomy and provide insurance." I shook inside.

"Bob, I will look into it," he declared as he hurried away.

The next day, the administration directed all students to begin supervised phlebotomy training. Insurance came later. Thank you Dr. Janeway.

Six months later I tested negative for HIV.

Chapter 11 – Medicaid Shenanigans

The triage phone rang in the pediatric emergency room. I was in the middle of my pediatric rotation schedule.

"Do you have any Tylenol? My child has a cold with a fever," came the mother's question.

"Yes, ma'am. Do you think your child needs to be seen in the emergency room?"

"Oh, no. She just has a cold, but I'm out of Tylenol." This caught me by surprise.

"Um, ma'am. Tylenol is available at your local stores. It will cost you $200 to be seen in the ER," I advised.

"Not for me. I have Medicaid. For us, it's free."

As a student, I oversaw triage for a bustling emergency room full of sick children. I had two of my own at home and considered my response.

"Ma'am, if you bring your child here for a bottle of free Tylenol, you will wait two to three hours to be seen. We will see you, but we will not give you any Tylenol. Goodnight." I hung up and peeked sheepishly at the attending physician who had overheard me.

"Nice job," he remarked with a smile.

We were all required to complete eight core rotations during our clinical third year: twelve weeks of Internal Medicine, eight weeks of Surgery, six weeks of Pediatrics, six weeks of OB/GYN, four weeks of Emergency Medicine, four Weeks of Family Medicine, four weeks of Neurology, and four weeks of Psychiatry.

Internal medicine covers numerous primary care areas in depth. Each organ system has a non-surgical specialist that is expected to know their focused area of expertise. There are neurologists for the brain and nervous system, gastroenterologists for the digestive tracts, dermatologists for the skin, cardiologists for the heart, infectious diseases specialists for all the germs and related illnesses, and more.

To be good at a specialty, a physician needs to learn everything -- from common to very uncommon -- in their narrow area of the body. They become experts with a depth of knowledge that is required when the rare, strange, or unusual presents. Family Medicine physicians need to know the most common twenty percent of diseases that occur across all specialties.

This scares some students. They are intimidated by the perceived amount of knowledge they must acquire. It is not more than any other doctor needs to know, and it allows us to see eighty percent of everything that walks in the door.

The more common diagnoses in each specialty are the ones seen by family physicians. As a result, primary care is the most diverse specialty with the best ability to appreciate the complex patient across all specialties. The more uncommon diagnoses are rare, and the system works well by referring the unusual to the specialist. They enjoy the challenges of the unusual and prefer to leave the common with others.

During the pediatric community care rotation at the Health Department in Winston Salem, NC, I found myself with a pediatrician and a pediatric neurologist who were evaluating the tiny child of a fourteen-year-old new mother. The child was losing weight, and a specialist was called.

The young mother and young grandmother watched. I conducted a careful medical history review of the mother and her child. I would need to repeat this to the doctor I was assigned to help. I was looking for the rare and unusual that would justify our neurology consult.

"Your child is losing weight. She has fallen off the growth curve for each of the last few visits. The doctors are concerned that there might be something abnormal going on. Have you noticed anything unusual, like fevers, or throwing up her food or diarrhea?" I asked, speaking to the older woman, even though the younger girl was holding the child.

"I am the grandmother. You should ask my daughter." I was a bit taken aback. The grandmother was twenty-nine years old. I couldn't imagine that teens had babies that grew up to have babies as teenagers themselves again. It was not in my experience base yet but was more common in the often-abused welfare system I would soon discover.

The state allotted resources to unwed mothers. Subsidized housing, food stamps, infant formula, and Medicaid were available. It made financial sense to have their children get pregnant as soon as possible to build a family with multiple welfare incomes. Marriage would negate some benefits, so the fathers did not marry their girlfriends. They lived next door in connected apartments and functioned as a family unit. They never claimed marital status so that benefits could continue. That was not a system I admired.

"Are you breastfeeding your baby?" I inquired of the young mother looking for any clue to unexplained weight loss.

"No. I give her the powdered milk and juice like I was told. And I feed her every two or three hours. She seems hungry a lot."

"What kind of juice do you give her?"

"You know, *juice*. Like Mom gave us. Dr. Pepper, Cheerwine, Mountain Dew…. you know, *juice*. But I dilute it half and half with water, so it isn't too sweet," she explained.

She stated that soda was what her mother had always called juice. Soda is cheaper than real fruit juice. By diluting it with water, she was starving her child. At her young age, this seemed logical. Sprite has lemons on the label. I was speechless.

After presenting my findings to the two attending physicians, they took over, and I watched as they arranged to admit the child to the hospital. The child would receive monitored feeding, and the family would receive classes on proper foods and feeding.

There would be lab work done to rule out infections and metabolic disorders, but the planned course of action would allow the child to regain lost weight and grow. Nothing unusual was found, and the pediatrician took over the case. Maternal education became the treatment plan and goal. In this case, Medicaid made a big difference, and the child and mother both benefitted.

Chapter 12 – Surgery

How do you spell abuse? S-u-r-g-e-r-y. My surgery third-year rotation would be incredibly demanding. Days started before dawn and sometimes, with evenings on call, lasted twenty-four hours. I had finished twelve weeks of Internal Medicine. It was October, and the surgery rotation would last eight weeks. I would be in the operating room with vascular, cardiac, general, and plastic surgeons, all showing off their specialty operative skills. The "scutwork" was relegated to the students. It was menial work no one wanted to do, like checking the labs, reviewing X-rays, drawing blood, and holding retractors in the operating room. It often involved running up and down stairs and walking long hospital corridors to get what we needed.

The benefit of our scutwork for the physicians was that they spent more time in the operating rooms. Surgeons seldom liked spending time in the clinic, but they enjoyed time in the operating theater.

My first full day on the general surgery rotation was disorienting. Patient rounds began at 6 AM. We had been instructed to be there early enough to know about the patients we would be visiting. As this was our first surgical rotation, none of us were sure of what we were supposed to know. Our resident physicians, from first-year interns to the fifth-year Chief Resident, would make regular demands of us. Their stated goal was teaching. Their other purpose, which often superseded teaching, was to make their own lives more comfortable.

"Ladies and gentlemen, welcome to your general surgery rotation. We need to get through rounds fast this morning, as I have a 7 AM surgery waiting," stated the tall salt-and-pepper haired, Senior Attending.

He appeared freshly shaved, and ready to conquer the world in his long starched white coat, draped over a baby blue button-down shirt and black-and-gold-striped tie. The other four residents watched intently and tried to look capable and informed. The two students, one of whom was me, appeared stunned and lost. That was expected.

We moved from bed to bed in a circular manner. Resident surgeons presented their patients to the attending, and a treatment plan was discussed or modified.

"Draw labs, order an X-ray, check a consultant's report, remove a feeding tube or urinary catheter, and get them ready for discharge," were our orders of the day.

The lowest ranking resident was a first-year intern. A few weeks ago, he was a medical student, and now his moniker ended with MD. He knew just enough to be dangerous.

"You students take notes of all the tasks due today, as we round. Make a list and split them up between you. We will meet in the Ward 5 resident lounge at ten this morning. Beep me if you have any problems," stated the intern. We nodded and walked away to get ready for the attending rounds.

The assembly gathered outside the surgery ward filled with patients. Attendings, residents, interns, and students formed an impressive gaggle. The fifth bed we came to held an elderly, gaunt man lying on his side and not moving. Our somber group of white coats gathered at the foot of his bed, while the attending removed and examined the chart hanging off the bed frame.

"I don't understand why this man is not getting better," he muttered for all to hear. "We removed his lung cancer completely, and he won't need chemo or radiation, yet he seems to be going downhill fast. Someone figure out what's going on here," he demanded.

The residents nodded and moved with him to the next bed. The ward nurses were standing by and listening at the front nurse's station as the procession moved on.

The surgeons all left. There were gallbladders to remove, and breasts to reconstruct.

I glanced at my classmate Susan and said, "I'll take the first five beds if you take the last four." She nodded and replied, "I have a long list for each patient. How are we going to get this all done by 10 AM?"

"Danged if I know, but let's get to work. By the way, did you get any food this morning?" I inquired, hearing my stomach grumble.

"Nope."

We moved from bed to bed, introducing myself. We wore the coveted short white coat of a medical student. We stuffed our pockets full of note cards and reference books that could help us navigate the new world around us. I had a shiny black stethoscope around my neck, and three pens in the left breast pocket.

"Hello Mrs. Sheppard," I said as I glanced at the chart retrieved from the foot of her bed. I'm going to take a blood sample to check your white blood count. This will allow us to see if the antibiotics are working well," I stated.

"OK. Do what you must. I think I've donated at least a gallon so far since I got here," she whined.

I moved the tray to her bedside and found the right color tube. I wrapped her arm with the thin brown rubber strap I had pulled from my left coat pocket. I felt for the bulging antecubital vein, cleaned it with alcohol, and blew on it to evaporate the alcohol. In went an 18-gauge, large-bore needle neatly into the middle of the bulge. Blood filled the tube all the way, and I sighed with relief.

We had many real patients to practice on during our last medicine rotation, and we had practiced on ourselves too. After my angry discussion with our hospital CEO following my HIV needle stick, we had all received phlebotomy instructions. Success was good, and the watching nurse smiled.

I sidled up to bed five, with the same older man in it, still lying on his left side, facing the nurse station and hallway. He had not moved. My instructions were to find out why he wasn't getting better.

I moved to face him. His eyes were closed, and he looked pale. Breathing came in shallow breaths.

"Mr. Stoneburner," I tried first without response.

"I am Bob Adams, a medical student, working with your surgeons." Then I said the one thing I knew.

"The operation went well, and you will be getting better soon." No response again.

The nurse came up beside me and asked, "Do you know that he is deaf?"

That startled me, and I replied, "No, I didn't."

I thought, and questioned, "Does he have any hearing aids?"

"Yes, in the bedside table next to his bed."

"Can you put them in his ears for me?" I requested uncertainly.

The nurse, grateful that someone on the clinical team had finally requested this, opened the drawer, woke our patient, and arranged his hearing aids with the volume turned up. She always did this when the family came to visit, but the morning rounds were brisk, and her input was rarely solicited. She usually just stood guard and watched the rapid progressions of surgeons, residents, and students.

As we were doing our student rounds, his family walked down the hall for their visit. Their mood was sad, as Granddad had been getting worse each day. They paused at the door at the same time the nurse completed her hearing aid task.

"Mr. Stoneburner," I began loudly. "The operation went well. We got all the cancer, and you will be feeling better real soon. We need you to start eating, so you can get out of here and go home."

His eyes opened, and he watched me with a new understanding and high interest. I repeated the same words, and he began to move. To our surprise, the nurse and I were swiftly surrounded by his family as they helped him sit up. They were all smiling.

"Granddad, you look great today!"

"Let's help him sip some water."

The wife squinted to read my name tag and walked over to hug me. "Doctor Adams, thank you for saving his life. We were worried, but now, thanks to you, he's better. Will he honestly be going home soon?" asked the family hopefully.

"Mrs. Stoneburner, I'm the medical student here, but the surgeons did get all the cancer, and there will be no need for more treatment. He should plan to get all better and go home soon," I said with a confident and happy tone in my voice. The family visibly wiggled, smiled, and murmured in delight.

The nurse moved away and watched my confusion and delight with an understanding that only a nurse has. Someone had finally summoned her for help, and the results were obvious. She and I would be accorded the family's praise and honor as part of the team that had saved his life. All because of the hearing aids.

He had grown up at a time when cancer was always fatal. In his heart, he thought that his life was done. When my white-coated visage stated otherwise, he woke up. He began eating, and the next day at rounds, it was decided he could go home the following day. No one on the surgical team asked what had happened. The nurse and I glanced knowingly at each other. The surgeons moved on to the next patient.

I would receive Christmas presents from the Stoneburner clan for four more years. They invited me to their home, nestled in the woods at the state borders where Virginia, Tennessee, and North Carolina came together. They wanted me to come deer hunting with them. I would be an honored guest for saving Granddad's life and cherish the turkey-call gift they sent me.

Their gratitude was embarrassing and humbling at the same time. Nothing I ever did or said ever changed their belief that I had been the "doctor" who had saved the patriarch of their family.

After many repeat invitations to visit, I decided to go and drove away for one weekend to a place few will ever see. Their neat country home was in the woods. The water came from a stream-filled cistern. The home's heat tumbled from a wood stove, and the cooked food emerged from a black-metal, wood-burning stove and oven. The vegetables came from their garden. The meat was squirrel, deer, and chicken, and the biscuits were homemade fresh at each meal. I learned gravy was to be poured over everything on my plate, and I gained five pounds.

I will never forget the perfumed air of fresh biscuits at 4 AM as the men rose to the hunt.

I did not get a deer.

Chapter 13 - Time Flies

One problem I noticed as a thirty-eight-year-old medical student was that I was sometimes older than my teachers. I had more life experiences, and they had more medical education. It turns out that the mixture of both is a powerful union.

I would go into an exam room with the doctor and find the patient talking to me. My hair was thinning with a hint of gray, and this was mistakenly interpreted as a sign of wisdom.

"Mrs. Phelps, I'm the medical student, here to learn. Doctor Knudsen is your doctor," I would instruct.

"Oh, yes, thank you," she would respond while glancing at the handsome man in the long white coat. Then she would turn back to me to continue the discussion. It irritated some of my teachers.

I only *appeared* wise. My ignorance would soon come to my home and scare my wife and me to death.

Weeks of surgery included leg amputations on sore-covered legs that smelled so bad we had to put strawberry odor spray on our surgical masks. Black toes with dry gangrene were amputated in people with diabetes. Black skin would peel away from the bone just by pulling on it. After dropping a forefoot and five toes into a waiting bucket yesterday, I decided to skip the surgery elective in our fourth year and add an obstetrics rotation instead.

Today was Friday, and the current surgical sub-specialty rotation had blissfully ended. It had been abusive and exhausting. I had spent the last eight weeks up at 4 AM, and home at 11 PM. The children were always asleep, so I would kiss their sleeping forms and tiptoe away.

This day had started as incredibly different. I had slept until 8 AM since the final morning rounds were not until 9 AM. I had seen my children awake and eating breakfast and had hugged everyone as I left.

Our evaluations were done, and I had passed, despite a genuinely unpleasant run-in with the surgical intern who seemed fond of telling us he was not "God." He was just "a god," and we should interact with him accordingly. Do what he said always, *do it twice, and never question him in front of others – ever.* His lack of people skills almost cost him a residency position in anesthesia. The Chief Resident advised me that he would not be welcome in surgery again. All had noticed his obvious failings.

Later that morning, I contemplated the previous seven weeks. There was a week of Ear Nose and Throat Surgery (ENT), scheduled as my final surgery rotation. ENT was last on the schedule, but I was exhausted. I went outside to eat my bag lunch and glanced up, for the first time in nineteen weeks, to see the sun. It glinted playfully through the bare branches of the tall trees.

I was stunned. When I started the surgery rotation, the trees were full of deep green leaves. Now the trees were bare. I had missed the Fall season in its entirety. Days consisted of walking to and from work, in the dark of mornings and late evenings. It pissed me off.

"I cannot settle for gray skies
when I have seen the sunshine.
I cannot enjoy concrete sidewalks
when I have met God on rocky trails.
I cannot leave you at a distance
when our spirits have embraced."
by Lisa Miller, my classmate

I ate my bag lunch and made a quick decision. It was time for me to act in defense of myself and my family. I dropped the crumpled brown bag in the trash and walk deliberately to the Chief of Surgery's office. When I got there, the secretary looked up and smiled.

"Can I help you?" she asked sweetly.

"Yes, ma'am. I'm Bob Adams, a third-year medical student. I have one more week to do in my surgery rotation. It is ENT surgery, but I can't do it as planned. I have a crisis at home, and will need to be gone next week," I stated inflexibly.

"Oh, I see. I will check with the Chief when he gets back on what to do," she replied with a bit of concern in her voice.

"Thank you. I'll be back in a week, and you can let me know then. He can fail me, or he can let me make it up in my fourth year, where I have electives. Either way, I am going home now. Thank you for your help." And I left the building, surveying the bare trees as I walked slowly and contentedly home.

I slept. When I woke up the next morning, my concerned wife was asking if what I had done would get me in trouble.

"I don't care. This is the time I need to rest and recover. An entire season has come and gone without me in your lives. I missed you and missed them. They've actually grown taller since I last saw them awake. It aches to know that. Let's spend time together with the children and be normal," I replied with determination. "I need that to feel OK again."

My wife, my partner, and best friend had always been there for me. Today was no different.

"OK, let's take the kids to Goofy Golf. That is something we can afford, and the kids love it," she smiled and reached for my hand.

"The crisp cool air is settling in
Fall is with us – quietly set upon us like
a mother pulling a child's blanket over her in her sleep.
Leaves falling in a flurry of yellow and red,
Sweaters, and mothballs, and the smell of new heat
Somehow balanced with that dread
of winters bleakness." by Lisa Miller, MS-3

The chilly winter week went by way too fast. On the following Monday, I reported to the Chief of Surgery's office to find out how much trouble I was in. The secretary expected me.

"Hi, I'm Bob Adams, and back from last week. Can you tell me what the plan is?" I asked courteously.

"Oh, hi, Bob. Welcome back. We have excused you from the ENT rotation, and you will not have to make it up. I hope everything at home is OK?"

"Yes, it is," I replied, pleasantly surprised.

"I think you are due at pediatrics at 8. Have a nice time," she smiled knowingly.

Chapter 14 - "Oh Shit!"

"Can you look at my throat?" requested my seventeen-year-old neighbor, who was standing in her grandmother's front yard next to ours.

"Sure, Elizabeth. Let me look," I responded with enthusiasm. The grass was fragrant and green, and the sun gleamed warmly on us. She was tall, blond, and cute as a button. I relished the opportunity to show off my skills.

"Open wide," I said and analyzed the back of her throat, which was coated with numerous thick, white plaques. The surrounding tissue appeared red but not swollen.

"Ouch. It looks like strep throat. You need to see your doctor. It needs antibiotics," I continued sympathetically.

It would not be my first or last erroneous diagnosis. She stopped by the next day to let me know that her doctor had made the diagnosis of mononucleosis, "the kissing disease," and she did not need antibiotics since a virus caused it. Oops.

I have not missed that classic presentation of "mono" since then. It is remarkably different in appearance than strep throat. I had simply never seen it before. I did not know what I did not know.

Later in that same month, my son reported home from elementary school with a sore throat. It was a Friday. My wife called and said Trey needed a doctor. As students, we did not have health insurance, but there was an area pediatrician that gave us free care when needed. I called their office and got an appointment. The diagnosis was strep throat, a common school illness. They gave him a liquid antibiotic and sent him home with a reassurance that he would not be infectious to others after one day on the medicine.

That night he still had a fever, and his tender, enlarged lymph nodes could be felt in the front of his neck. We gave him the medicine four times a day, exactly as prescribed. He could not eat because he felt horrible all over, and it hurt to swallow. Popsicles were better tolerated. He was not getting better, and swallowing the medicine was becoming difficult. *Did my dirty germ-covered white coat bring germs home?* I wondered. *Of course, it did.*

Sunday morning began as an actual rare day off for me, and Trey was having more trouble swallowing the liquid medicine. His neck appeared more swollen. We were both concerned.

"We should take him back to the doctor today, and let them take another look," I pronounced.

We drove three blocks to the doctor's office. It was Sunday, and they only had morning hours. There was another doctor there, alone, to see the walk-ins.

"Sir, my son was seen two days ago, and today he can't swallow the medicine and has a fever. His neck is more swollen," I said concerned. Jeri watched.

He glanced at the chart and said, "He has strep throat. This is not uncommon. You need to keep giving him the antibiotics," he stated with conviction. He was busy, and he moved to the next patient.

We were getting free care, and this prompt dismissal intimidated me.

Sunday was a tough day and night for us. We could not get him to swallow the medicine, and his neck and throat were so swollen that, by the evening, his tongue stuck out of his mouth so he could breathe. His breathing was labored. He could not lie down because of secretions, making him cough with pain. I wanted to go to the emergency room, but I feared that doing this would be viewed negatively by the doctors we had already seen.

We waited until morning and took turns sitting up with our son. He had to lean forward to breathe, and drool covered his shirt front. Swallowing was impossible.

I was off to school early, and Jeri agreed to go to the pediatric office again at 7 AM and wait to hope someone came in early. The doctor arrived at 7:15. He recognized Jeri and our car. It was the only other car in the parking lot, so he walked over curiously. Our son was in the back seat, and the back door was open.

"Hello, Mrs. Adams, how is your son doing today?" he asked warmly, approaching the car with a friendly smile. He shook her hand and peeked in the car at the young form leaning forward in the back seat.

His face froze.

"Oh, shit!" he gasped. The child he saw was a pediatrician's worst nightmare. He knew immediately that Trey's condition was serious and life-threatening. He had a retropharyngeal abscess that any experienced physician would recognize as a surgical emergency. The pus pockets expanding in his neck needed to be drained, or the infectious pus could erode into a vessel, causing total body sepsis and death. Children hardly ever survived if it happened.

"Mrs. Adams, please do not take your son out of the car. I will have him seen at the ENT surgeon's office right away. His condition is dangerous, and he needs surgery," he announced with fear in his voice.

He pulled out his cell phone and called the office of Doctor May, the Chief of ENT surgery. His secretary answered, confirmed he was in, and told him to have Trey come directly to his office. What she did not say was Doctor May was already in the first surgery of the day. It was 7:30.

Jeri did as she was told. It was a short four blocks to the Wake Forest School of Medicine, and she knew where to park. Doctor May's office was easy to find. For the last two years, she had wandered these hallowed halls with me.

The Chief of ENT Surgery had a brightly lit corner office on the second floor. The secretary expected her and informed her Doctor May would be up as soon as he finished the surgery that he was currently doing. She smiled reassuringly but looked concerned when she saw Trey. It was 8:00. Jeri beeped me on my call beeper, which displayed her location. I was needed and made a quick exit from the ward where I was working. I ran to the office.

At 9:30, Doctor May walked into the room wearing green surgical scrubs. He was smiling and had his hand out to me.

"Hello, I am Doctor May," he intoned pleasantly and glanced over at our child sitting in a wheelchair, leaning forward, and drooling into a small towel.

"Oh, shit!" he said as he let his hand drop. He went into emergency mode and scared us both with a series of quick instructions.

"Bob, you know where the CT scanner is. I want you to take your son there now. They'll do a CT of his neck. Bring the films with you to the operating room admission area. They'll be expecting you, and we will go into surgery to drain an abscess in his neck," he directed.

To his secretary, he said in a commanding, staccato voice, "Ellen, call the OR and tell them we're coming right now. Tell the anesthesia staff that shift change is on hold. Have them ready when we arrive. Call the CT scan staff and tell them to get anyone on the table off of it, and we are on the way with an emergency. Bob, you and your wife, go now," he finished.

We left for the CT scanner in a hurry, with wide eyes, and I heard him say determinedly to his secretary, "Ellen, when you talk to these people, remind them that they all owe me favors, and I am calling all those favors in, right now!" He sounded very concerned. It did not calm us.

As we approached the CT scanner on the first floor, the double doors were being held open by a doctor and a technician who were looking with curiosity at what might be coming. They ushered us to an empty scanner bed.

"Does your son need sedation, or can he hold very still for a few minutes?" whispered the doctor.

Trey heard the question and stuttered a wet reply that he would hold still. We lifted him onto the cold, hard, movable table and placed a rolled towel under his neck to help him breathe. The scan took one minute.

A few minutes later, the radiologist came into the room with the wet 2-by-3-foot films. He held them up to the overhead lights.

"Oh, shit!" he mumbled and gave them to me.

"Get going, and good luck," he said as he handed me the bare films. Off we went to the surgery suite down the hall. My hands were shaking.

Again, the doors were held open, and the staff was waiting. We were waved to a table where the anesthesiologist stood with a needle in his hand. It connected to an IV bag, and as soon as it was in and running, Doctor May appeared in clean scrubs.

"We will be in the operating room for about forty-five minutes. I'll come to talk to you both after we're done. You can wait in the waiting area," he directed calmly. He turned and rushed away to follow the bed, now rolling rapidly away.

Two and a half hours later, he came into the waiting area. His scrubs were soaked with sweat to his belly button level. He looked tired.

He sat down with us. "Your son had an abscess that had dissected deep into the tissues of his neck. Tracts of pus were going everywhere. It was the worst I've ever seen, and the surgery was difficult. But I think we got it all."

"Due to the swelling and difficult surgery, we will leave him intubated and neuromuscular blocked. He'll be in the pediatric ICU for a few days," he finished.

Trey's bed burst through the door on the way to the ICU upstairs. He had a large breathing tube in his mouth and other tubes everywhere. I was petrified, and Jeri was mute. We thanked him and rushed away with my wide-eyed wife to follow our son. I was just a frightened father now.

The next few days would change me forever.

Chapter 15 - Oh My God

The next day began with Jeri and me holding hands protectively over the inert body of our son. Machines were keeping him alive. We had constantly whispered to him. "You are strong. We love you and are so proud of you. You will feel great when you wake up."

"What are you going to do?" we had learned to ask the nurses. There had been a series of questionable decisions made affecting our son's care. It had been twenty-four hours since the surgery. As a student, it was our job to check X-rays after intubation to make sure the tube was in the right place. If it were placed too far down, it would go into the right main bronchial airway. It would deny air to the left lung, which would collapse on itself.

The morning after surgery, I went to look at his chest X-ray and was astounded to see the tube was indeed in the right main airway. No one had checked. It appeared, to my inexperienced eyes, that the left lung had collapsed.

I asked the radiologist on call to look, and he uttered, "Oh my God." He called up to the pediatric ICU and spoke with the nurse, who called the doctor on call. That resulted in a quick response to pull the tube partially back out until breath sounds could be heard on both sides. Another X-ray was ordered, and a series of orders were written to increase the respirator pressure PEEP (Positive End Expiratory Pressure) and add bronchial dilating medicines to the routine every two hours.

A quick explanation and quiet apology were given. We were not happy.

We resumed our watch and noted his heart rate was increasing, but I could hear breath sounds on both sides now with a stethoscope I borrowed from a nurse. The left side was faint.

I watched the overhead monitor in our private room, and the heart rate had climbed to 200. It was due to the albuterol - asthma inhaler - they were giving him regularly. At midnight, the nurse came in and began to give another dose of albuterol. I requested her to stop.

"His heart rate is too high to give that medicine now," I stated with certainty. "Please don't give it." Jeri nodded in support.

"These are the doctor's orders for tonight. What do you want me to do? Wake up the doctor?" she queried in an irritated tone of disbelief.

"Yes, please, ma'am, I wish the doctor would come see my son."

I did not know it at the time, but we had the legal right to refuse treatment. The nurse frowned and left the room.

When the doctor on call came into the room, I pointed out the heart rate and my concerns about giving a drug that would make it faster. He agreed.

"And, sir, I wish you would look at his arms and legs. They're quite swollen."

"Well, Bob, that is common, because of all the IV fluids we're giving him. Don't worry." And he left.

Unconvinced, I left Jeri in charge and started research on my own. I reviewed his lab work and saw his sodium levels were quite low, and the urine specific gravity was also very low. He had gained four pounds of water weight. It seemed like "SIADH" that I had learned about, and I recalled it was quite dangerous. It could cause the brain to swell, and it always caused the edema I was concerned about.

"System Inappropriate Anti-Diuretic Hormone" secretion had many causes, and it made the body swell. I started looking for causes. Nothing I read seemed to apply to my son until I stumbled on a paragraph that reported it was seen in ventilated patients when the air pressure was set too high.

Trey's PEEP (Positive End Expiratory Pressure) was set at the maximum recommended level since they were re-inflating his left lung. It had been going on all day, and both lungs were clear. I found his nurse and told her of my concerns. She refused to call the doctor again, and we felt helpless.

The next morning, as doctor-rounds approached, I stood bedside and waited. When the doctor arrived, he was in a hurry. He had lots of patients to see. I blurted out my rehearsed research findings and requested that the PEEP be turned down. Third-year students (rightfully) have little credibility in the ICU. I was thanked and reassured, but they made no changes.

I was a father first, so I rechecked my medical facts and waited. The doctor would come back. The nurse was sympathetic but not convinced.

When he came back later that morning, I was waiting. We had more time now.

"Sir, respectfully, my son has had his right mainstem bronchus intubated, which collapsed his left lung. The on-call doctor last night canceled the medication that had his heart rate over 220 after I requested him to. His PEEP is set high, and that may cause SIADH. I know this is unusual, but his lungs have clear breath sounds bilaterally, and I would appreciate it if you would turn down the PEEP pressure. He's swollen all over, and his urine is inappropriately dilute. Please?" I pleaded.

The pediatrician listened but was not convinced. I was a medical student and had limited credibility, but was also a parent, and I might be right.

He nodded and reached for the chart to write the order to reduce the PEEP. He did not seem convinced or happy.

"Thank you, sir," I mumbled. "We will be here all day, monitoring him."

During that day, my mother and younger brother arrived by plane from Virginia to help at home. I had called them in a helpless panic, and they came without hesitation. By 11 PM, I was tired and needed to go home to check on our daughter. I kissed Jeri, who was "on guard," and went down to our ancient Chrysler Town & Country station wagon.

It was dark out, but the car was distinctive. All four tires were different. We had bought them, one at a time, by getting discarded tires and patching them for $2. Sitting quietly in the driver's seat, I searched for the keys in my pocket and tried to find the ignition. My hands were shaking, and my breathing came in choked sobs. I could not start the car, so I sat there, wanting to let it all out. I needed to cry but was not sure how. The pain in my chest needed release. One tear and one sob found voice. I took a few deep breaths, found the keyhole, and started the car. The radio blared. I drove slowly home.

This tale ends happily, with our son released from the ICU after four days. My mother and brother had provided comfort and care for us all.

It was the beginning of Christmas vacation for our children's school and me. We would be a family again and help him heal together. His swelling resolved, his voice returned, and he ate ice cream. Doctor May had saved his life with immediate action. With Christmas a week away, I would be with family during the daytime again. Brother Bill and Mom returned home. Their generous help had proven invaluable. Their gift of self will never be forgotten.

From that day forward, I walked into the house, removed my germ-covered white coat, threw it in the washer, and washed my hands. The stethoscope was cleaned at work with alcohol swabs between patients. No kiss *hello* was permitted until the washer top closed.

The next month, a ten-year-old arrived in the emergency room with the same condition. An experienced physician had identified it immediately. Alas, before the needed surgery could happen, his abscess eroded an adjacent vessel. He became septic and died.

This experience profoundly moved me as a father with a critically sick child. My son and namesake had come as close to death as he could and survive. The emotions of fear and helplessness stay with me in my memory always. It made me a better physician when dealing with the inevitable losses my patients would experience in the years to come.

Chapter 16 – Breech Delivery

My favorite rotation, so far, was obstetrics at the nearby community hospital. I found myself one evening under the tutelage of a Family Medicine resident doing a fellowship in complicated obstetrics. He was learning to perform surgical Cesarean section deliveries. He planned to practice in an under-served area near his birthplace in the mountains of Tennessee.

"OK, Bob, the labor deck is full tonight. We have eight in active labor. I plan to deliver every baby that comes out above the waist, and I expect you to deliver the ones that come out below the waist. Is that OK with you?" he asked, smiling.

He was doing a fourth-year fellowship in family medicine with obstetrics to qualify for high-risk obstetrics and surgical C-section deliveries. His home in rural Tennessee had fewer doctors than were needed, and they were located far apart. Family Medicine doctors in underserved areas often required to do their own Cesarean section deliveries. This evening he was in the operating room, and I was on the deck to catch all the vaginal births I could. There was a board-certified obstetrician somewhere, but I had yet to see her.

"Yes, sir," I replied expectantly. This was a student's dream come true.

I wore a clean set of green doctor scrubs and my student white coat with pockets stuffed with the tools of the trade this time, including a stethoscope, reflex hammer, penlight, antibiotic manual, and obstetrics pocketbook. The coat would come off when we got down to the baby delivery business, but it would not be far away. The information I sometimes needed was not in my brain yet. It was in my pockets.

The baby catching business was usually pretty simple. But when something went wrong with a delivery, it was often unexpected and critical. Nature had given women the ability to have children at home, and in the woods, and in the middle of nowhere since time began. I needed to play catch and wait for the placenta to follow.

Live, healthy births in the United States have always been distressingly fewer than in most of the world. Mothers and babies still died in childbirth. I knew that but was unsure why. Drugs, alcohol, smoking, obesity, sexually transmitted diseases, inadequate prenatal care, teenage pregnancy, and diet all played a part.

Today, all was going well, and I was smiling.

"Ok, Linda," I crooned to the fourteen-year-old soon-to-be mother, "let's have another push when you see the contraction on the monitor." She felt nothing because of an epidural line dripping anesthesia into her spinal area. It made it more comfortable, but hard to use the muscles needed to push.

Her mother stood at the head of the bed and watched with an anger she had already made clear.

"Do not give her any anesthesia. She's fourteen years old and having a baby. I want her to feel every damn contraction." She had declared as we were checking her in.

I had nodded and mumbled, "She's not a minor now under the law. I will ask her what *she* wants." Epidural it had been.

The head of the baby protruded halfway out, and there was no need to cut a surgical episiotomy to make room. It would be smaller than the average baby. She smoked cigarettes, like many of her friends in Winston-Salem, NC, the home of R.J. Reynolds Tobacco Company. Mr. Bowman Gray, Sr., as past president of Reynolds, had left money in his will that the family would use at his request to move the medical school here from Wake Forest, NC.

I placed my hands on the baby's head and tried to control the progress, as nature pushed the head out. It emerged through an expanding vaginal canal covered in clear, leaking, amniotic fluid and blood. Once the head popped out, the rest was automatic. Out slipped the neck, shoulders, and body into my waiting hands. I sat on a stool, dressed in a blue paper surgical gown, wearing sterile gloves. My legs were spread in case my slippery bundle was to wriggle past my hands and into my lap.

I cradled the small child in the crook of my left arm and reached for the two clamps needed to be placed on the blue, pulsing umbilical cord. Once clamped, the nurse handed me scissors, and I cut the cord, which was trying to slip away from me.

"It's a girl!" I declared cheerfully. This was amazing. I was present as a new life entered the world. The new mother's mother scowled, and the young girl gazed down excitedly. I handed the baby to the nurse and tugged gently on the cord to encourage the placenta to follow.

"Bob, you better hurry up over there," offered my mentor. He was leaning against the door of another room and peering in at a woman in labor.

"This one is coming soon, and if you don't want to watch it hit the floor, you better get here fast," he chuckled.

The placenta began making an appearance now, so I reached inside the newly enlarged vaginal opening and pushed fingers up into the uterus, traced the edges of the placenta, and eased it gently out into the stainless-steel bowl held by the smiling, but bored, nurse. She had seen it a thousand times. A quick inspection revealed no tears or missing parts. The placenta appeared completely intact, so I was free to move on. If a piece of the dark red pancake-shaped placenta, covered on one side by blue bulging veins, was missing, I would need to reach back inside, find it, and remove it. This would avoid dangerous post-delivery bleeding — but not today.

With the placenta, umbilical cord, and plastic clamps in the bowl, I stood up as various fluids dripped down my gown onto the floor and my paper-covered sneakers. I handed the bowl to the nurse and moved eagerly to the room where the resident leaned casually against the doorjamb.

"Do I have time to change my gown and scrub up?" I asked.

"I wouldn't if I were you," he purred in a warning and expectant voice. I entered the room where a nurse stood between the legs. She moved aside and opened a new set of sterile gloves for me to slip on. I removed my used ones and reached out, one hand at a time, while I watched the bulging area between the soon-to-be mother's legs present a pale mass of baby.

My new gloves were on, and the nurse moved the stool to where I needed it. I sat down, excited and hopeful. The senior resident looked bored and moved on. He thought his job was done.

The monitor registered a big contraction, and the nurse continued to coach.

"OK, sweetheart. We're almost done here. Let's have another good push," she encouraged.

A groan came from the woman I had yet to meet, and a baby started to emerge. I followed protocol and placed my hands on the presenting part to control the descent. It was soft. This was not a normal texture, so I scrutinized suspiciously. There was a crease in the presenting part. Oops. It was not a head I was holding.

I gaped with wide, panic-filled eyes at the nurse and said, "please go get that doctor back here immediately. We will have a breech delivery here soon," I directed in distress.

"Ma'am," I tried to direct calmly, "do not push again. Your baby is coming out butt first, and I need you to hold on for a minute."

I had no idea what I was supposed to do next.

Chapter 17 – Twelve-hour Surgery

I am always pleasantly surprised when professional dealings on behalf of my patients allow me to meet a happy surgeon. If they are happy in their chosen profession, they are caring and understanding with the patients I send them. If they are unhappy, for whatever reason, I routinely need to apologize for their rude or inappropriate behavior.

Surgery is a challenging and demanding profession. It requires an intimate knowledge of anatomy and all its variations. Hands and eyes must work together with patience, care, and precision. One microscopic wrong movement can sever a barely visible nerve, vessel, or organ. The need for a surgeon is often both urgent and critical.

A life may depend on the surgeon's skills. As a result, the life they often lead is one of high stress, limited sleep, unexpected demands, and new anatomic discoveries that challenge their abilities. The result is often an unhappy and acutely stressed doctor that would rather be on one of their two sailboats than in the hospital once again. They must deal quickly with a patient they just met, or tell a family waiting outside that they had failed.

I enjoyed surgery and have always been in awe of the willingness of a person to allow a physician to cut them open, wander around their insides, alter their anatomy, or remove the offending tissue. But I determined early in my surgical rotations that I would never make an excellent surgeon. I lacked patience.

"Just cut it," I would think to myself as minutes turned into hours. The surgeon I was assisting continued to separate one tissue layer after another while hunting for the offending organ, vessel, or abscess.

"Dang, why don't you cut it? My hands are going numb holding the retractors," I whispered.

"That is your job, Bob. Pay your dues now. There will be more fun stuff later," observed the surgeon.

The excellent surgeons, the ones that loved to come to work, would show me, one layer at a time, why they could *not slice and be done.*

The great ones knew the diagnosis before the CT scan would confirm it. They could sense an appendicitis or hidden abscess from across the room. They had a sixth sense, based on years of doing the same thing for hundreds of patients, which made them invaluable. The older doctors relied on experience and the learning that occurred bedside.

Aristotle was their hero. There were no MRIs or CT scanners or ultrasounds when physicians a century ago had to make decisions. They relied on the skin and eye color, fingernail deformities, skin's salty taste, and even the sweet taste of urine to make various diagnoses.

Breath's odor could diagnose diabetes, a throat abscess, or multiple systemic disorders. Today's older doctors rely on experience and are almost always right.

When a scan or lab could not define an abnormality, the older doctors were often summoned. They would ignore the CT, hold the patient's hand, listen to their breathing, gaze deeply at their eyes, sniff the air, feel under skin creases for lumps, and ask about other symptoms. A headache would take them down one path, and frequent stooling patterns or gas pains, down another diagnostic path.

"This patient likely had a case of acute appendicitis yesterday. It has ruptured now. As you note, she has a new fever and a lack of pain. She needs to go to the O.R. right away," he would state confidently. No one ever questioned him. He was always right in these matters. The nurse was already on the phone to the surgical suites to reserve a room. He would save the patient's life today.

During my vascular surgery week-long rotation, I found myself in the operating room with our renowned chief of the service. He was scheduled to replace the abdominal aorta, and both connected femoral arteries, with a polyester Dacron graft. The surgery was expected to last twelve hours.

My job was to hold retractors. I would hook the heavy, stainless steel L-shaped devices, with handles on my end, to the edge of the patient's wide-open abdomen, while the knife-master precisely dissected down through layer after layer to find the bulging aneurysm threatening to rupture.

A symphony of movement supported his every action. Anesthesia monitors displayed the patient's vital signs, oxygen saturation levels, and respiration rates. The anesthesiologist stood at the top of the bed, monitoring it all and watching the sedation medications drip steadily. Machines breathed mechanically for the patient.

There were two medical students, a resident surgeon, and two surgical nurses dabbing and passing instruments in support of the primary surgeon. The circulating nurse moved around softly, placing a Lifesaver or lemon drop in each team member's mouth to keep calories circulating. She would squirt a bit of water in our mouths to keep us hydrated. The attending surgeon rarely looked up.

I needed to pee. There was no way I would last a few more hours. I had passed my retractor to the other student and had stepped back. I could see even less than I could before. I pondered what to do and needed to ask permission to be excused. The surgeon had an unpleasant reputation for the treatment of residents and students. I waited for an opening in the action and rehearsed in my mind what I would say.

I remembered that, by protocol and definition, below the level of the table was to be considered not sterile. We were all wrapped in our sterile gloves and scrubs, but our shoes and below-table-clothing were deemed to be *dirty*.

A lull occurred right after the surgeon asked for another 3-0 gut suture.

"Doctor Osterman, may I please be excused? I need to use the bathroom," I whispered.

He did not look up, and his response was abrupt. "I've been here for ten hours. You can be here ten hours."

I had expected his response and had readied a comeback.

"Yes, sir." I turned toward the nearest nurse and followed resolutely with, "Nurse, please place some towels at my feet. I am going to pee now." The room seemed to stand still for a second, but the surgeon glanced up at me with a bit of wonder in his eyes.

He peered back down and grumbled, "Fine. You are excused for five minutes."

I smiled to myself and moved smoothly away. It would be longer than five minutes before I returned. Sometimes it was valuable to be older and have life experiences under my belt.

Chapter 18 - Why I Am Not a Pediatrician

A young couple, with their one-year-old son, presented to the emergency room concerned about their ill-appearing child. He had been correctly diagnosed with an ear infection two days before and placed on age-and-weight-appropriate antibiotics by their pediatrician.

He did not get better. He got worse, with more crying, less eating, and today he had a fever of 103.5 but was quiet. He did not respond to light, noise, or tactile stimulation. The emergency room pediatrician was instantly concerned.

"I need a blood count, a cath urine, and an IV right now," he told the nurse. She moved to comply as the concern in his voice spoke volumes. The parents looked on, wide-eyed and confused.

After the IV was placed, blood drawn, and a catheterized urine sample sent off, the physician ordered high dose IV antibiotics to be given STAT. We waited for the needed lab results. He directed me to get a mask and sterile gown on. He did the same.

"We need to do a spinal tap to rule out meningitis," he told the parents. "Why don't you two have a seat in the waiting room, and we'll come get you soon. I'll admit your son to the pediatric ICU as soon as we're done here."

The next day, on morning rounds, they informed us that the child had been diagnosed with the extremely dangerous bacterial meningococcal meningitis. The spinal tap had confirmed it. The infection had started in the ear.

This morning, only hours after he had come to the emergency room, the child was being kept alive by machines. He was brain-dead. The parents were bedside, and in shock, as the ICU pediatrician once again outlined his findings.

As a group of students, we were all stunned and confused. *"How could this happen? Did someone do something wrong? Is there a reason for it?"* we all wondered in dismay.

There were a few more tests, and a neurology consultation to measure for brain activity. And finally, a determination that these parents had lost their first-born child to an ear infection gone bad.

Later that day, after local family members had come to be with the child, the parents gave permission to disconnect their son from life support. I stood behind the mother, who cradled her son in her arms, with her lips caressing his pink, warm cheek. Her young husband held her free hand and tried to stifle sobs as tears rolled down his cheeks. The room was cold and brightly lit.

The pediatric resident-in-training was tasked with removing the endotracheal tube and turning off the respirator. She cried quietly as she performed this final task. I surveyed the room through my own tears. The entire entourage witnessing the tragedy displayed their distress with tears - except one.

The attending pediatric physician stood aside, in his starched white coat with a neatly tied tie and monitored the proceedings. He was dry-eyed.

That was the moment I knew -- I could never be a pediatrician.

Chapter 19 – Dermatology

I love dermatology. The smartest few in medical school fight for a residency in this specialty, since dermatologists are well-compensated, with almost no middle-of-the-night emergencies.

There are few residencies in dermatology available, so competition creates the resultant selectees as top-of-the-class students. Often, women get these slots, since it is easier to raise a family in a specialty with regular hours and no night emergencies.

Eczema, dermatitis, fungal infections, skin cancers, and many more skin conditions often point a doctor towards another related medical condition. The skin is the only totally visible organ system in the body. It gives us clues to look somewhere else.

"If it's wet, dry it. If it's dry, wet it. But, for God's sake, don't touch it." That is the standard joke about how to survive a dermatology rotation.

I am examining the hands of a thirty-year-old male. There are serpentine, raised, pale lines on the backs of both hands. They have been there for weeks. They don't itch or hurt. It looks like worms have been carving tunnels under the surface of his skin. His medical history is negative for other symptoms, new medicines, supplements, or any other clues.

I summarized the exam with the attending physician.

"That sounds like you have a case of granuloma annulare. Let's go take a look," he responds. "I can make that diagnosis from across the room."

We make it to the patient's room, and my attending stops at the door. The patient has his hands on the knees of his blue jeans.

"Yep. Granuloma annulare. Look it up," he says sympathetically. "I will be in my office."

I have made the same diagnosis many times over the years. Once you have seen this, it is easy to recognize. Nothing else looks like it. It will often go away without medications. Steroid creams and injections, and ultraviolet light therapy help. Freezing the lesions with liquid nitrogen (like we would treat a wart) often stimulates a remission.

As a resident, decades ago, we often ignored this self-limited skin eruption. Today, with better pathology and infectious disease diagnostics, we know the condition is associated with tuberculosis, schistosomiasis, syphilis, and other infections.

Decades later, my office visit began with, "Doc, I have a weird rash on my hands. The urgent care doc told me it was granuloma annulare," began my forty-five-year-old patient, holding out his two hands.

"He is right," I followed assuredly.

"I did some Google-reading, and it says you can treat it with liquid nitrogen like you did that thing on my back last year. Can you do that again for this?" he requested.

"I've never tried that. Usually, I use steroid creams or injections, but we can try it if you like," I answered.

For three months, he returned every two to three weeks, and we applied liquid nitrogen to the squiggly lines on his hands. There was a definite improvement, but we were not winning the battle.

He was frustrated, and so was I.

"I will send you to a dermatologist," I remarked after we had discussed the lack of progress.

The biopsy report, by the dermatologist, came to me as well. The patient had syphilis. This sexually transmitted disease caused his granuloma annulare, and if I had looked more thoroughly, I would have seen the same lesions on his arms and legs.

"I know what I did, Doc," he whispered. "I shouldn't have done it," he finished.

There was no reason to explore his embarrassment any further.

"The health department will follow you for now. They'll treat your contact too. I expect the hand lesions will clear up with the treatment, so that is one thing we won't have to worry about. I'm sorry I did not think of getting a biopsy sooner."

He nodded in understanding. Sexually transmitted diseases are increasing in older populations, including nursing homes. Immunizations are helping with hepatitis B, and the cancer-causing infection: human papillomavirus.

It is easy to forget about these infections when taking a patient history. Asking about sexual behaviors often reveals surprising and useful information.

Penicillin was discovered in 1928. It was used to cure syphilis worldwide. Without treatment, the infection will take over the body and brain.

From 1932 until 1972, the U.S. Public Health Service provided free medical care to 600 men and women with syphilis in the impoverished town of Tuskegee, Alabama. They were enrolled in a study and given free burial insurance and treatment for *bad blood.* The doctors did not treat these patients with newly available antibiotics.

The investigators did this to find out what would happen to a patient with this progressive and disabling infection if it went untreated. They watched while it progressed to stage-two and stage-three syphilis. Stage-three included brain infection. The researchers discovered much and documented it all while they allowed the disease to progress.

In 1997 President Clinton formally apologized for that unconscionable experiment by government doctors.

Chapter 20 - Summer Army Rotation

Military medical school scholarships paid a monthly stipend that was half of a 2nd Lieutenant's starting salary. They also provided for one month of work on active duty, drawing full pay. That month, in our third and fourth years, allowed us to do rotations in military hospitals where we might want to be selected to do our residency.

The best Family Medicine residency was at Madigan Army Medical Center, Fort Lewis, Washington. I went there for both third- and fourth-year rotations.

"Lieutenant Adams, you were here last year, and we liked you. You should be going somewhere else this year," stated Colonel Thompson. He was the Department Chief.

"Yes, sir. I know, but I liked it here last year, and I want you and your staff to know that when I fill out the required five choices for my residency, it's going to say: 1. Madigan, and 2. through 5. will be: *Kill me, kill me, kill me, kill me.*"

This earned me a nod and a smile.

"Bob, I have to be honest with you, your Part 1 board scores are not that great. We have lots of applicants for our program. Why would we choose you over these other applicants?"

I was prepared for his question, as it had come up before.

"Sir, our Parallel Curriculum study program is different in preparing for the Part 1 standardized exam. We're more clinically oriented from the start. There's less rote memorization of test facts. I admit that I will not be the smartest doctor you bring here, but I will be the best doctor you graduate."

"Good answer," he stated with a smile.

I spent the next four weeks doing family medicine, obstetrics, and pediatrics with the family medicine staff. I made sure they knew of my intent, but I needed insurance.

I went to the nearby Hood Canal on Saturday, with rented scuba tanks, to catch much-loved Dungeness crabs. I knew where to go. I had done some diving there the year before. Usually, I would never dive alone, but this spot was only 15–20 feet deep, and I could walk into my secret hole from shore. I drove my car there and made the dive. I had a mission.

"Sir, during our orientation, you said that if we students had a problem, we could call you directly," I began with concern in my voice. Colonel Thompson was on his home phone.

"Yes, of course, Bob. What is your problem?"

"Well, sir, I seem to have a cooler full of fresh-caught Dungeness crabs, and I have no place to cook them."

A brief pause followed, and my future Department Chief responded. "I see, Bob. And what time may I expect you?" he finished with a bright smile in his voice.

We had a delightful dinner of crabs and beer, and I got the residency I wanted.

"Doctors will have more lives to answer for in the next world than even we generals."
Napoleon Bonaparte

ARMY RESIDENCY – BACK IN UNIFORM

Chapter 21 - Graduation at 40 Years Old

The Wake Forest University graduation speaker was following a routine he had followed before. There were families of over one hundred doctors and two hundred lawyers looking on expectantly for his words that would lend credence to the vast expenses they had shouldered to add MD or JD to their family member's names.

Row upon row of black-robed men and women layered the chairs in front of him. The rows behind them were filled with wide-eyed family and friends that hoped these new graduates would achieve their dreams. That journey would begin now.

Jeri and our two young children sat in the back rows, with other expectant families representing our class. They were smiling. I sat in the front row wearing a soft black robe, adorned by a purple and gold James Madison University MBA collar, and the longer Wake Forest doctorate hood in gold and black. It was a good day.

Four years in the making, our graduation ceremony was a fun but brief moment in our lives. Pictures were taken, and families smiled, but few would ever look back on that time again. It was a start, but the finish was years away. Doctors and lawyers would need to complete internships and residencies. These jobs would pay poorly and require years of long, exhausting ordeals in the trenches of libraries, offices, hospitals, and clinics. Families would endure it with them.

"Take a look at these rows of graduates. There are two lawyers graduating today for every doctor that walks across the stage. That's because for each doctor we graduate, we need one lawyer to sue him and one to defend him," began the guest speaker. His opening line drew appreciative and entertained giggles from the crowd. Some in the crowd remained silent. They were the doctors that already practiced medicine and mourned the truth in that jest.

I found the entire event unique, necessary, and boring, but it included a commission in the U.S. Army Medical Corps as a Major. It was one of the reasons I went to school on a military scholarship. I wanted to rejoin the forces of the U.S. military, wear the uniform, carry a green ID card, and stand at attention in the evening when the bugler sounded 'retreat' as the flag was lowered. I missed the brotherhood and sense of mission that came with all that.

My decision to go to medical school followed my transfer from active service to the Reserves. This allowed me to train monthly with a SEAL Team. I could parachute, scuba dive, blow things up, and stay in shape on weekends while pursuing other careers or schooling. It was a time when war was uncommon and unexpected, so I sought my fortune elsewhere in the business world.

No one slapped me around when I chose to leave active service. No one made me look ahead or begged me to stay. The military forces were drawing down in size.

I quickly learned that the business world did not give employees free health care and thirty days of annual paid vacation. Employers did not offer a raise when you got married, or another one if you had children. Life insurance was not subsidized, and taxes were higher.

After a few months of working menial jobs for less than my previous housing allowance had been, I began to reassess my choices. When I asked my younger co-workers about their plans for their futures and they just looked confused. Their plans went as far as next weekend.

I got on the phone and called the Navy. "Take me back, please. I want to serve again," I asked various contacts from my recent past.

"Lieutenant, we appreciate your interest, but the military is reducing its force size. We don't need more frogmen now. Stay in the Reserves, and we'll call you if we need you," was the consistent reply. *Oops.*

I went back to school for an MBA to obtain money from the GI Bill while drilling monthly with the Teams in Little Creek, Virginia. I earned enough to live and eat.

Then I fell in love.

I was unaware she was my soulmate, but my future wife knew. The day we met, I was trying to sell her something in a new business I was starting. I had come to her home wearing a coat and tie and met her and her sister. They shared an apartment. Her beauty rattled me, but I got her phone number.

After I left, no sale made, she turned to her sister and said, "In case you want to know, I just met the man I'm going to marry."

Today was graduation day, and she sat in the audience, with our two squirming children, now six and eight, and watched the next phase of our lives together begin.

Chapter 22 – Intern year – No Sleep

"Doctors carry around their own personal graveyards," stated my animated attending physician when I lamented the preventable loss of a patient. "That graveyard follows us around tapping on the subconscious. It keeps asking us the same questions."

"Is there something we did wrong? Was there something else we could have done?"

These soul-searching questions surface too many times in a physician's life.

There are also grateful smiles and warm hugs. The birth of a first child. The fear and faith in a child's eyes. The grateful parent. The ultimate trust of another human being. All other forms of happiness pale in comparison.

The Army paid for school and gave us a small cash stipend to live on, but it was not enough for a family of four. So, we graduated in debt, like everyone else. For the four years of school, our car had been worth what I could get in scrap metal for it. The tires were all worn and different.

Graduation came with a medical degree and an officer's active duty commission. Residency awaited, and I would wear an Army uniform at Fort Lewis in Tacoma, Washington. We were going to travel by car to Madigan Army Medical Center.

A family cross-country trek was ahead, so we tried to buy our first new car. We wandered into the Plymouth dealership in Winston Salem, NC, and found a brand-new Plymouth Voyager van. I filled out the paperwork, noting we had no assets, a $50,000 debt, and little income. We explained to the salesman that the following month would begin my new career in the Army as a doctor. We nervously hoped for the best.

When he returned, after discussing our application with his finance manager, he smiled warmly and gleefully said, "The manager simply wants me to find out how many vans you want."

The trip was an adventure, and it followed a meandering path from national park to national park. We crossed the Rockies and stopped to sing 'America the Beautiful' while admiring the 'purple mountain majesties.' We carried personal items that could not be trusted to the movers. We slept in the cheapest tolerable hotels that allowed a dog. Our black spaniel-mix took it all in stride.

Graduation was on 5 May 1991. My first day on active duty again would be 1 July. In those seven weeks, we traveled across the country, found an affordable house within a safe distance to the hospital, and settled in. The closeness was essential, because I would be driving home sleep-deprived most nights. We set a ten-minute limit on drive time from hospital to home. The house we found was eight minutes away. Reasonable.

Intern year began with long days and longer nights. Rotations in each specialty were exhausting, with overnight call every second or third night. Those nights on call seldom allowed for sleep. Obstetrics, general surgery, internal medicine, and family medicine inpatient services were the most demanding. I did not come home often during those months, but when I did, I slept hard. Weekends and holidays were rare.

I had served eighteen years in the Navy, active and reserve before the new Army adventure had begun, so I knew my way around a military organization. In the first week of July, after orientation, I walked into the Residency Director's office and submitted leave (day off) requests for Christmas Day, New Year's Day, and a few other key holidays. The director's response noted that the days I had requested were already federal days off. I remarked that I had a family, and if he approved these, I would not find myself on call those days, stuck in the hospital. He smiled, admiring my wisdom, and stamped them *approved*. I could always cancel the request if I got lucky and had the day off anyway. Experience came in handy.

Most new doctors were commissioned as Captains. As a Major, one rank higher, I could get things done with less hassle. My rank had been calculated by giving me half credit for prior commissioned years served. It resulted in a higher graduation rank and a higher starting salary. *Thank you, Uncle Sam.*

On-call nights in the hospital were always frantic. The beeper went off frequently, and I would run from lab, to ward, to bedside, repeatedly all night. At home, the children wondered where Dad was. My wife realized there was a way to answer their questions that would help us all. One night she showed up with our two children and a picnic basket containing dinner.

It became a tradition. We would set up in the ward lounge areas, lay out dinner on available furniture, and eat together. The beeper would sometimes pull me away, but I would return to eat and hug the family goodnight. It sent important messages to all: *Dad is working, and he loves you.*

Chapter 23 – The Salmon Are Running

I have always been a fisherman, and I love the rivers, the watery hunt, and the delicious trophies. Washington State is crisscrossed with streams full of salmon and trout. There seems to be a fresh run of some species of salmon each month all year long. That drove my wife crazy at times when I wanted to explore another stream on a rare day off.

By Christmas, I had settled into a consistent routine of clinic, hospital wards, and long call nights. I had made friends with more senior residents who liked to fish, and they had taken me to a little-known spot on the Nisqually River that flowed right through our Fort Lewis Army post.

It was a ten-minute drive from the hospital to the mouth of a chum salmon fish hatchery. The hatchery-raised salmon returned in large numbers in December. They stacked up at the same place each year, and if you knew where this was and could walk the trails to the bend in the river below the hatchery, you could catch your limit of two large salmon quickly.

I kept a cooler and a rod in my car rigged and ready. In December, when I was in the clinic, I would meet with the front desk staff and tell them I had moved my last appointment of the morning and my first appointment of the afternoon, to other places in my schedule. This opened up thirty minutes and gave me ninety minutes for lunch. As soon as I could, I would leave, in uniform, and drive to the river trail. There I would put on chest waders over the uniform, grab my rod, and walk the path to the sweet spot. I often went alone and would use newly learned techniques to hook and fight a couple of large salmon to the bank, drag them back to the cooler, and return on time.

If someone went with me, we would take pictures of our trophies. I posted one such trophy-shot on my office door. The next day, after the morning clinic, the Residency Director summoned me to his office.

Lieutenant Colonel Wayne Schirner was a kind and caring teacher. He sat me down and said, "Bob, it's fine to have fun during your intern year. But, since it's my job to work you hard, it isn't a good idea to advertise the fun you're having. You might want to take down the fish picture on your door." I did.

My patients always applauded my efforts to get away and do something more rational than working all day every day. They would see the other resident physicians and me in various states of exhaustion. We were assigned to the clinic following our ward time in surgery, obstetrics, emergency medicine, etc. Most of these rotations were inpatient, all-night-call months.

These long work hours would severely tax our mental abilities to the point that we would experience real difficulty making our thoughts and speech logical. Madigan Army Medical Center was the biggest and best medical center in the Army inventory. Army physicians of great renown staffed it. Patients fought to be seen there or have their babies delivered there. Our services were free to the military, their families, and retired military in the area.

When we showed up, pale and exhausted, the patients sympathized. If they had needs that we could not address, they knew we had other resources at our disposal. They were our patients and we were their doctors. It was a team learning experience, and we all benefited.

I took my responsibility to assigned patients seriously. They trusted me, and I knew I lacked enough experience to deserve that trust. I would often lie awake at night, thinking about an unsolved medical presentation. I frequently needed a test result or advice from a specialist before I could tell my patient what their problem was or how we would fix it.

"Doc, I'm coughing up blood again," whispered my sixty-four-year-old patient. She was a lifetime cigarette smoker and knew it could be serious.

"What do you mean by *again*?" I asked.

"Well, I went to the ER last month with a cough and told them I saw blood in my sputum. They gave me antibiotics and sent me home. It seemed to help the cough, but I see blood most times when I cough now." She seemed more curious than concerned.

My mind went to *cancer* right away, as that would be the worst possibility. I stayed calm and reviewed the many other causes that included infection, tuberculosis, bronchitis, or a foreign body. The list flowed through my mind, and a careful exam followed.

"Your lungs have wheezing that seems to mostly clear when you cough, but not completely. You don't have a fever, and you took ten days of antibiotics, so let's get a chest X-ray today to make sure we're not missing something." She appeared relieved with my proposal. After we were done, she went to radiology for her X-ray, and I moved to the next room, where a child with ear pain waited.

It was 5 PM, and my clinic was over. I needed to get upstairs to the ward where the patients we had admitted were waiting for the night crew to arrive. As an intern, I would be busy all night, and the day team needed me up there to pass care responsibility of their patients to our night team so that they could go home.

I glanced at my computer and noted a few lab and X-ray reports were ready. The X-ray was from today's clinic, so I paused to read it.

"Mrs. Salerno, this is Doctor Adams at Madigan. How are you?" I asked calmly.

"It's bad news, isn't it?" she responded. "You wouldn't be calling me with good news."

This caught me by surprise, as she was correct. "Well, yes ma'am, I'm afraid the X-ray shows a large area in your right lung that is suspicious for cancer," I stated sympathetically, and then I paused.

"It isn't like I didn't know it, Doctor. I've been losing weight too," she replied.

I kept quiet as she continued. "It's sad too because I have just received a large settlement from a car accident last year that was not my fault. But I guess my children can have fun spending it," she finished with a resigned sigh.

The rest of the conversation is lost, but it is similar to many others I have had. I always offer hope that it isn't cancer, or if it is, we will treat it and make it go away. Her tumor was large, and the bleeding meant it involved her bronchial tubes. This was not a cancer we could likely beat.

My father had died at sixty-three and I was learning that it was the age most smokers died. I felt defeated, made a note in her chart, signed out of the computer, and hustled to the elevators that would take me to the medicine wards upstairs.

Chapter 24 – Orthopedic Emergency

My first trauma case as a new MD was on the orthopedic service. I had seen plenty of trauma as a medical student, but this would be my responsibility now. I was an intern, and our emergency room was routinely dealing with broken bones from pediatric falls and vehicle collisions.

My signature line ended with MD, but I was not yet licensed by any state to practice medicine. The emergency room patients did not care, and the Army gave us six months to pick any state to apply to. It would be good anywhere we practiced in the military network. Pennsylvania only charged $100, so many of us used this cheaper option to obtain a license.

"Bed three. Motorcycle crash with a severely broken leg needs you now please," began the ER nurse when I arrived at her station in response to her beeper summons.

I moved quickly and with anticipation to bed three. A nurse was holding the hand of a twenty-two-year-old soldier wearing blue jeans that had been cut along both sides to his groin on the right leg. His face had abrasions on the same side from his chin to his forehead, and his right eye was swollen but not shut.

There was a damaged leather coat, gloves, and helmet on the floor. He appeared in pain but alert. The reason for the pain was evident at first glance. Halfway between his knee and his foot, the leg was bent about seventy degrees away from straight. The foot and lower leg were lying on the bed with the foot pointing in the wrong direction. It looked like he had two knees – one where it was supposed to be, and another one halfway down his lower leg. The foot was a grayish-blue color.

I looked at the nurse first. "Corporal Ball was brought in by ambulance a few minutes ago following his motorcycle crashing into a pickup truck on post," she began. "His vitals are stable, and despite some obvious abrasions, there's no active bleeding. His head and right shoulder hurt but the leg hurts much worse. I have a wet towel with ice on the way," she concluded, looking at me expectantly.

"Thank you."

"Sir, I am the ortho doctor on call today, and I need to check your leg. I need to know if you can feel me touch your foot and see if there's a pulse." He nodded.

I lightly touched his cold foot and felt for a pulse on the top of his foot. Nothing.

"Can you feel me touching you?" I asked. He nodded yes, and his eyes showed pain.

I checked another place for a pulse without finding one. This was not good. If we did not get the blood flowing to his foot, he could lose it.

"Did anyone page the resident on call?" I said to the nurse.

"We called him first but were told he's in surgery, so we paged you."

"OK. I'm heading to the OR to talk with him, and I'll be right back. Get the ice and towel on it for now, please."

"Yes, Doctor. Do you want to order any pain meds?"

"When I get back. I won't be gone long. I need to talk to the boss," I said over my shoulder as I hustled quickly toward the elevator.

I put on a paper mask and booties and walked into the operating room where my senior resident was. He was lit by the glow of a large surgical light over the table, and his nurse was dabbing at some blood dripping from his patient's knee.

"Sir, I need some help in the ER. I have a motorcycle accident patient with a closed tib-fib fracture at the mid-leg level, and no pulse felt in his foot," I stated quickly.

"I am operating. What do you need?"

"What am I supposed to do, sir?"

"Do you remember your basic anatomy?" he asked, looking up at me.

"Yes, sir," I gulped.

"Well, go back down there and put the leg back the way it's supposed to be." He looked back down.

Is that all the guidance I'm going to get? Well, I guess he thinks that's all I need to know. And I can put it back the way it's supposed to be, I thought, while moving slowly and reluctantly toward the door.

I paused. "Should I give him some pain medicine first?"

He looked over his mask at me with a twinkle in his eye and said lightly, "Would if I were you."

"Nurse, what do we have here for pain that I can give now?"

"We have morphine."

"Good. What's the most I can give in a single dose?" I whispered.

"Usually, it's ten milligrams."

"OK. Please go get that and give it now. I am going to pull his leg back in line."

She nodded with slightly wider eyes and rushed to the meds room. On return, she had a bottle in one hand and a syringe in the other filled with ten milligrams of morphine. I inspected the container and confirmed the dose.

"Please give that right now. I confirmed that he has no allergies to meds." The patient was watching with interest.

"Corporal, once the medicine takes effect, I'm going to pull on your leg and get your bones back where they're supposed to be. The morphine will help a lot, but it's still going to hurt. I need to do this to get the blood flowing back into your foot." He nodded and was already showing signs of sedation with his eyes fluttering a bit.

His eyes closed, and his breathing included a faint snoring sound. I looked over at the nurse who was waiting expectantly.

"Please grab his thigh and keep him from sliding down the bed. I'm going to slowly pull on his foot and move the bones back in place." The nurse nodded and took a towel and threaded it under his thigh, grabbed both ends and held tight. She had done this before.

I wrapped my hands around his cold ankle and pulled away and downward.

A growl began in the patient's throat and grew to a moan. I felt the bones touch as I quickly realigned them. The moan became a guttural scream, and his eyes flapped open. This got all eyes in the room looking our way. The bones popped into place like pieces of a jigsaw puzzle as I held on to the ankle. The scream stopped. I was sweating profusely and so was the nurse.

"Done. Let me check for a pulse," I mumbled. "Got one," I said, smiling and grateful.

"Let's put some ice on this for now, and we can make him a nice temporary splint, get an X-ray, and let the boss decide if he'll need surgery or not."

"Nice job Doctor," smiled the nurse.

"Um, Doctor Adams, since you're here, could you look at a four-year-old in bed ten? We paged pediatrics, but they'll probably call ortho anyway. We think he has a dislocated elbow."

"Nursemaid's elbow?" I asked with interest.

"That's what we think. The dad pulled him up by his arm at the playground, and he hasn't been able to move it since."

"Absolutely. Let me check him."

I moved to bed ten, met the dad, and solicited the same story. His son was sitting quietly and holding his right arm slightly bent at the elbow. No sign of pain now, but it hurt if he tried to move it.

I had seen this and fixed it a few times before. It is common in children that are lifted by their arms quickly, by well-meaning parents. I explained this to them both and told them I could fix it quickly with their permission. The dad said, "Yes please."

'Son, I want to hold your hand for a minute. It won't hurt." I said softly. He nodded but looked scared.

I lightly grabbed his wrist and slowly rotated it such that the hand was palm up. I placed my other thumb on the radial bone head where it came into the elbow and put slight pressure on it.

"OK. Let's move your arm slowly toward your face," I said encouragingly as I slowly bent his arm. I had their full attention now.

"Ouch!" yelled the boy with new tears forming in his eyes as I felt the radial head pop back into position. I let go as the boy pulled his arm back, and I watched him slowly straighten it without pain. Then he tried to bend it and was surprised to feel no pain again.

"Well, all better," I announced with glee. Dad looked amazed, and the child appeared surprised.

This was starting out to be a very good day.

Chapter 25 – Should I Worry About Ectopic Pregnancy?

Late in the evening, I found myself on the ward analyzing the labs of the patients our team was managing. Our attending physician sat next to me. He was ultimately responsible for our actions and decisions related to the care of our hospitalized patients. It was also his license we operated under. We had MD after our names, but we were interns with little experience. We had been medical students a few months before and were still learning the trade we were now tasked to practice.

I received a page on the digital beeper on my belt. It was from the triage nurse, asking me to call a patient. I glanced at my watch and saw it was almost midnight. The triage nurses took care of all routine patient questions and needs. It meant something more important was going on.

I picked up the ward phone and called the number on my beeper.

"Hello?" came the calm voice of the woman who wanted a doctor.

"Hi, Mrs. Williams. This is Doctor Adams. I am the on-call physician tonight. How can I help you?" I asked, sounding as competent as I could.

"Oh, hello, Doctor," she replied. "I called because my period has not stopped. It usually lasts six or seven days, but I'm still bleeding, and this is day seven. I don't know if I should be worried or not," she stated evenly.

I thought protectively about the time, the symptoms she was worried about, and the differential list of diagnoses I might have to worry about. Nothing terrible came to mind for a woman that was on the seventh day of seven days. Certainly, she was not in any danger tonight.

"Ma'am, it seems like this could be of some concern if it continues, but we will know better tomorrow if the bleeding worsens. It seems OK to wait and see. If you bleed more heavily or have any bad pains, please call me back, but I think it's OK to wait and see," I responded as confidently as I could.

"All right, Doctor. Thank you for calling me. I appreciate your time," she said gratefully. She hung up, and so did I.

As I sat there contemplating the conversation, a thought hit me.

I turned to Doctor Gilliam, sitting next to me. He had heard my end of the conversation but was lost in his chart review. "Doctor Gilliam, I wonder if I should worry about an ectopic pregnancy in a woman who's still bleeding on the seventh day of what's usually a six to seven-day period." His response was measured and direct.

"Bob, in my experience, if the thought of ectopic pregnancy ever enters your head, you need to rule it out." He went back to his chart.

With a moment to digest his advice, I picked up the phone and dialed the same number. It was late. I was unsure, but I needed to know more.

"Hello?" came the sleepy reply.

"Mrs. Williams, this is Doctor Adams again. I'm sorry to bother you, but after discussing your symptoms with my attending physician, we think it would be best if you came in to see us for an ultrasound. It's unlikely, of course, but we need to check you for an ectopic pregnancy," I said apologetically.

"Of course, Doctor. I'll come in. And thank you. The fertility doctors warned me about that possibility when they reattached my fallopian tubes."

Light exploded in my brain. I had not thought to ask about risk factors.

She showed up, as instructed, at the radiology department, where we did a directed ultrasound with the help of the radiologist on call. The ultrasound findings were distinct, definitive, and concerning.

I scrubbed in with the obstetrician, who then removed the fallopian tube bulging with a pregnancy. It might have killed her if it had ruptured.

I have never failed to consider ectopic pregnancy since.

Chapter 26 – Admit Periorbital Cellulitis

The beeper paged me to the emergency room five floors below. It was lunchtime, and I had not finished the notes from morning rounds. This was why we were here, but it was a bother. Rather than calling, I took the elevator to the ER and found the doctor that had paged me.

"Thanks for coming," the attending emergency room doctor said. "There's a peri-orbital cellulitis patient in the ENT room for you to admit. Please do it quickly. I need the room." He saw me nod, so he walked away.

I thought about what I would find and walked to the room where the patient and his wife waited. They knew that I was coming and understood they might spend tonight in the hospital.

I introduced myself to both persons and began an exam. What struck me directly was that his red, swollen eye socket and surrounding red tissue did not look like what my inexperienced brain thought would be periorbital cellulitis. Something did not seem right. Even his age was wrong. Periorbital cellulitis is more commonly a pediatric diagnosis, seen in children under eighteen months old.

I wanted some help. I found the number for the ophthalmologist on call and dialed his number. I presented the case, with the physical exam, current labs, and presumed diagnosis as made by the ER physician. I noted that, in my opinion, it might be something else and wanted his help.

"Did you get a CT scan?" he queried.

"No, sir," I responded.

"Please get one and call me back if they find something," he said and hung up.

Lunch was not going to happen now. I dialed the radiologist and explained I needed an immediate CT scan of my patient in the ER. There were now two more senior physicians pissed off at me.

The ER attending wanted the room and demanded I admit the patient and get the CT scan from the wards. The radiologist did not want to stop his busy workload to scan a likely soft tissue infection just to please an ophthalmologist that was too busy to see the patient.

"Doctor Adams, I need you to admit this patient. I have another patient I need to see in that room," demanded the senior ER doctor.

"Sir," I started delicately, "I'm not sure this is cellulitis. I've asked the ophthalmologist to see him, and he needs a CT scan before he will come. I will need to leave him with you until we get the CT results."

He was not happy, but I knew if it was something eye-related, this patient did NOT belong on an internal medicine ward. He might need surgery. I went back to the elevator and could sense the laser heat of an angry doctor burning two holes in my back.

An hour went by, and my beeper went off again. It directed me to call radiology.

"Hello, Doctor Adams," began the kindly voice that answered. "I wonder if you could come down to the CT room. I have something to show you," he finished in an almost apologetic tone. It was the same angry radiologist I had imposed on earlier.

I went there straight away. The radiologist smiled meekly and wanted to explain what he saw on the CT scan. The patient had a large abscess behind his eye that was eroding into the bone and pushing the eyeball forward. This was a surgical emergency and needed speedy surgical attention.

I called the ophthalmologist with the CT results, and he beat me back to the emergency room. My gut had proven right. He did not end up on the medicine ward, getting antibiotics that would have done no good. Instead, the patient went immediately to the operating room, where he did well. *Whew.*

Chapter 27 - He Chose to Die

A senior attending physician summoned me to his office for a patient he was seeing.

"He has shingles involving the trigeminal and ophthalmic nerves," he started. "I'm concerned about his visual symptoms, and I want him admitted for observation."

Shingles? I wondered. *This is not a condition requiring admission to the hospital.*

When I suggested we might handle his case as an outpatient (and avoid adding one more patient to our busy inpatient service), he reminded me angrily, and in no uncertain terms, that his patient was to be admitted immediately.

"Yes, sir," I responded dutifully and moved out to begin the paperwork. The patient was in the exam room, waiting for me.

He was seventy-two years old and fit. His exam was perfectly normal except for the glaring red, raised blisters on the side of his face. This typical, angry, shingles rash began at his ear and wrapped around to his nose and eye on his left side.

"Does it hurt?"

"Yes, sir. It hurts a lot. That is why I came in today. Nothing is helping the pain," he answered.

"The nurse will bring you up to our hospital ward, sir," I finished. "I'm heading up there now to get your orders done for an MRI scan of your head, shingles antivirals, and some pain medications."

It was easy and routine. I had no concern at all. His doctor wanted him watched, and his brain scanned, so off I went to accomplish the plan. No problem.

The next day he worsened. He showed signs of neurologic impairments affecting his vision. He had new balance issues and had fallen while trying to go to the bathroom. His left neck and left cheek had new dark purple bruises around the shingles blisters.

The MRI scan suggested that a virus might be affecting the brain. It would have access via the ophthalmic nerve of his eye. This was unusual. We were not sure what to do, so I called Infectious Diseases to help.

We increased medications to destroy the herpes zoster (shingles) virus. Pain medications were given by IV, and he could rest.

The next day he could not walk. His legs were weaker, and sensation in his feet was markedly decreased.

As the weeks went on, his symptoms increased and worsened. We had multiple services involved. Nephrology was watching renal failure. Neurology was monitoring the brain and lower extremity weakness, and physical therapy was working on the legs. An infectious disease specialist was dealing with the shingles virus in the brain and a new fungal infection in the throat and esophagus. His immunity was also impaired.

We brought the family in to discuss his code status and help them write a living will. The progression of his symptoms had been unexpected.

Six weeks passed, and we had won. He was alive and able to eat soft foods again. But he was paralyzed below the waist. It had been a long, hard battle, but there was a future now.

We began discharge planning with the patient and his family. He would go from here to a rehabilitation facility. They would help him learn how to use a wheelchair and learn how to catheterize himself for bladder emptying. We discussed skin care and muscle wasting. It would take time and a multi-team care effort.

Saturday morning, I came in early for patient rounds. His bed had been moved to the nurse's station.

"He wants to talk to you," began the nurse. "There are new developments, and he's refusing his food and pain medications," was all she would say as she spun away.

"Doctor, I wanted to tell you this personally. I know how hard you all have worked for me. I appreciate it more than words can describe. My family and I have discussed it, and they agree with me."

"Agree with what?" I asked, not sure where the conversation was going.

"Thank you for everything. But, sir, I am done now," he stated softly, but inflexibly.

My eyes widened and filled with tears. *Was he telling me he was choosing to die? Is that even possible?*

"No. You can't do that. We're ready to discharge you. We won. You are better," I pleaded.

"Doc, look, before this happened, I was joyfully walking the local streams daily, catching trout and salmon for dinner. The quality of life waiting for me now is unacceptable. The cost and strain on my family is not something I'm willing to put them through."

"I want you to let me go," he finished.

What? You can't do this. We saved you. Nothing going on now will kill you! After all our work to save you, you want to die!?

He could see me struggling, but he held my hand and closed his eyes. The nurses were watching.

I stood there a few more minutes, holding his hand and watching him breathe comfortably. I looked around for help - anything. There was none, so I squeezed his hand and moved on.

"He can't do this, can he?" I asked our attending physician when he came in.

"Of course, he can," began my kindly mentor.

"We don't make decisions like this for the patient or his family. It isn't uncommon for a healthy husband to die soon after his life companion passes. We have more control over life and death than our books lead us to believe. Talk to him if you can but respect his wishes."

He died four days later. I tear up as I write this feeling like I should have done more.

His family sent me a sincere thank-you card containing a copy of his obituary. Their hand-written note thanked me for allowing him his choice and his dignity.

The obituary revealed a fantastic story of an accomplished sailor who had served his country for almost four decades. I wish I had talked to him about some of that. I had no idea.

Chapter 28 – I'm Sorry

After an exhausting four weeks managing the sickest patients on the internal medicine ward, I was blessed with an outpatient neurology rotation. The days started at 8 AM and ended at 5 PM. It was a glorious break from the long hours of inpatient ward work.

On the wards, I had often been awake for twenty-four hours or more before signing out to get sleep. Sometimes I would be back the next morning to find a nurse waiting for me to correct an order I had written in my sleep-deprived state.

"Doctor, you did not mean to give this patient that dose of medicine, did you?" she would ask sweetly.

I would look at an order I had written in a handwriting I barely recognized and responded in horror at my mistake, "Oh my God, no. You did not do that, did you?"

"No, sir, of course not," she would respond, smiling. "Please fix that order for me," she would smile. The nurses had been there longer than we residents-in-training had. They knew to protect the patients and us from the abuses we endured while working 36-hour shifts.

Today was different. We conducted morning rounds in the doctor's lounge as we studied relevant learning cases from the day before. After rounds, we were given a day of clinic outpatients to see, evaluate, and treat. Each patient would be reviewed with the attending physician if we encountered any difficulty.

My day was going well. I was learning about migraine headaches, peripheral neuropathy, and brain pathologies. It was refreshing.

"Oh, no. It's her again," an attending physician said, as he studied the next patient due to be seen. "Give her to the resident, please. I will be in the break room." He walked away, and I saw the front desk lady look at me sympathetically.

I walked into the exam room with a smile and my hand out. She shook it quickly because I would not put it down. Touch is an essential part of my intent to connect with patients. But, before I could finish introducing myself, she launched into an angry and frustrated summary of her medical condition. She had nerve pain in her leg that was excruciating and would not go away. Medicine was not helping. I was the fifth doctor she had seen.

"No one will help me," she screamed. I could see the staff moving away from our room as I closed the door.

"Please start over at the beginning and tell me about your pain. I will try hard to help," I said kindly.

She paused suspiciously but started at the beginning. She told me she had undergone a cardiac catheterization over a month ago, and after the procedure, she began having burning pains shoot down her leg. They started near the site where the catheter needle had been inserted and ran down her leg day and night. It was worse if she bent over or climbed up stairs.

She had asked the cardiologist if the procedure could have caused her pain. They had quickly and collectively denied it was the reason. They referred her defensively to neurology to determine the cause.

It was now my task. I thought about the anatomy of the leg and remembered the past cardiac catheterization procedures I had seen. It seemed to me, most likely, that the catheter needle had struck the femoral nerve which ran along the vessel they were working in. I could not envision another explanation. It seemed like everyone was trying to avoid blame.

I did a careful and complete neurologic exam as she watched me with a vigilant and suspicious glare. Her demeanor was angry. I thought about what I would say.

"Mrs. Ronthal, you are completely correct," I stated authoritatively. "It is likely that the cardiologists hit your femoral nerve during the heart catheterization procedure. That explains the pain where you feel it." I had her complete attention now.

"The good news is, when a nerve is injured like this, it's almost always a temporary condition, and it should go away completely in a few months. As you noted, your pain is less this week than it was last week. It will continue to improve until it's gone," I finished in my best professional voice.

"How long will this take?" she queried.

"It could take up to six months, but each day will be better than the day before, and the medicines you're taking will help," I concluded.

"I knew it. Thank you, Doctor," she blurted out as she reached out to hug me.

I smiled and probed, "By the way, Mrs. Ronthal, has anyone said to you they were sorry?"

"No," she paused.

"Ma'am, on behalf of all your doctors and Madigan Army Medical Center, I am sorry this happened to you. And, I am sorry we had not said that before now," I stated formally, as I stood up.

We chatted a bit more, and she left with a smile. Her limp was noticeably better. She went to the front desk to check out and was laughing with the receptionists. The attending physician poked his head out of his office at the laughter.

"What did you do? I have never even seen her smile," he asked me as he dared to walk the halls toward me.

I told him about my conclusion. "And I finished by telling her we were all sorry. That had a profound effect on her pain and her perception of pain."

He nodded pensively. We both smiled.

Chapter 29 - Munchausen's and Seizures

"Doctor Adams, your favorite lady is back. Bed three," announced the nurse.

"Is it Mrs. Allen?"

"Yep, and she wants to see a surgeon for her abdominal pain. We did a CBC and a metabolic panel already. The results are both normal. Time for you and your magic again."

Mrs. Allen was a regular visitor to our emergency room. She has had every part of her body scanned or X-rayed. She has had unneeded surgeries, and she is taking medicines that are of no value to her. She has Munchausen Syndrome, named for Baron von Munchausen, who was well known for embellishing stories of his life.

Mrs. Allen's psychiatric condition was perplexing, and I consulted our department chief after her last ER visit.

"What can I do for her?" I wondered out loud in frustration.

"Bob, there's no treatment that I am aware of for this condition. If you can get her to agree to see a psychiatrist, they might find out what her stresses are and perhaps get her to look at herself differently. This is a lifetime condition. We have little to offer her," he replied.

I moved to bed three, wondering how I would get her to go home again. I pulled the curtain back and watched her face change from normal to a distressed expression. Then she looked at me through squinted eyes. She recognized me, and her face returned to normal.

"Oh, poo, it's you. I'm not going to get anything tonight, am I?" she whined.

"No, ma'am. Not tonight," I noted with conviction. Usually, the acting continued or worsened until she got more tests or drugs.

"Your lab tests were wonderfully normal, and I'll ask the nurse to give you a copy with your discharge paperwork. OK?"

"OK," she replied in resignation.

"When's Doctor Adams not here?" I overheard her ask the nurse.

"Oh, he's a resident doctor, so he's almost always here," came her calculated reply.

"Damn," she whispered.

The next day found me back in the ER for my day shift.

"Doc, we have a seizure in bed one."

"Got it. Get me ten milligrams of Valium and meet me there," I replied.

I rushed to the bed to find a woman with a grand mal seizure. Two medics were holding her arms and head so she would not fall or hurt herself. I got ready to help her, as I had been taught. Valium given IV would help her almost immediately.

I saw her look at me through rapidly blinking eyes, and then look upward again. This was not something a person with a seizure would do.

"Here is the Valium, Doctor," said the nurse.

"Wait on that for a moment, please. I need to check something. Let go of her right arm, please," I directed and moved to where the medic was. He stepped aside, looking confused.

"I need to check her arms first." I picked up her right arm and held it over her face. Then I dropped it. She was still shaking all over, but the hand fell to the shoulder, missing her face. Then I picked up her other arm and repeated the test. The arm fell to the side again.

"I will not need the Valium, and you can let go of her head," I said to the nurse and watching medics.

"Ma'am, you can stop your seizure now. I won't be giving you any medicine today," I stated loudly.

The shaking continued, but I saw her eyes find me again.

"No drugs today," I repeated kindly and decisively.

She stopped shaking.

It was a rehearsed method used by drug seekers, and it frequently worked. In an emergency room, standard procedure was to treat seizures rapidly with high doses of narcotic drugs. Her eyes gave her away. They should have stayed invisible and rolled upward.

"To confirm the fake nature of her presentation, all I needed to do was drop her arm on her face. If it had been a real seizure, the hand would have hit her face. She avoided that discomfort by moving the hand away from her face," I explained to the medics after directing the nurse to discharge her.

"If you look in her records, you will see a pattern of drug use and abuse. You will also see that she has done this before, and she got the drugs she wanted. We put a flag in her chart, and we told her that we did so, but she'll try again here or at another ER," I explained to the medics.

I was pleased with myself, and the medics were impressed. I swaggered with an unappreciated and inappropriate arrogance back to the workstation.

Chapter 30 – Eleven-Minute Vasectomy Champ

As a medical student I was taught how to perform a surgical vasectomy. The procedure was simple. But, to do it well, the surgeon needs to identify and isolate the vas deferens (spermatic cord). It feels exactly like a firm spaghetti noodle and is also about as slippery as one.

The cord passes through the prostate gland and hangs loosely in the scrotum attached to the testicle. Like the testicle, it floats around the scrotal sac and moves with the testicle when muscles pull it up or down to adjust to temperature changes.

It is a brilliant design and function that keeps the sperm at a comfortable temperature. Too hot and the sac elongates to cool things. Too cold and the testicles and all the surrounding parts head north and tuck themselves up inside the warm pelvic spaces.

I had assisted with my own vasectomy one afternoon as a student two years earlier. We had done about six vasectomies in a row. I was assisting the physician. The more we did, the easier it seemed. I had been putting it off for a few years, and my wife wanted to come off birth control pills.

"Hey, do you mind if I hop up on the table and you do me next?" I asked the doctor.

This request caught him by surprise, but when he realized I was serious, he suggested we do lunch first. I joined him back in the procedure room an hour later, wearing a surgical gown.

The procedure involves a local anesthetic injected into the skin of the scrotum. Then the vas deferens is manipulated until it is pushed tight against the numbed skin. While holding it tightly in place, with thumb pushing it up between two fingers, a special clamp is used the grab the slippery *spaghetti noodle*. That is the hard part, but once in the clamp, the skin can be opened with a tiny incision through which the cord can be grabbed and pulled out. We tie one or two sutures on the cord. The cord is cut, and each end is cauterized to scar shut the tiny central hole that would have allowed the sperm to pass.

We then allow the cord to return to its floating home. The single-cell living organism we call sperm is produced by the millions daily. If not used for reproduction, they die and are chemically reabsorbed. The same is true of all the cells in our body. They are continually being used, die, and replaced.

"I want to help with my vasectomy," I laughingly told the doctor, "It will make a better story when I call my wife tonight."

I was already numbed and sitting up watching his handiwork.

"All right. You can tie one of the sutures if you put on some sterile gloves," he responded, shaking his head with a smile. He paused to grab a pair of rubber gloves and tear open the package.

I put on the gloves and held my hands up like a surgeon in the operating room. When the time came, the doctor held up one end of my newly severed vas deferens and handed me a nylon suture. I wrapped it neatly around the presenting part and tied a perfect square knot. He cut the loose ends, cauterized them, and dropped it back into the tiny hole.

As expected, Jeri did not believe me when I related the story that night.

Two years later, I was the resident doctor, and my current urology rotation was designed to expose me to various urology surgeries. It involved time in the operating room for complicated surgeries involving the bladder, ureters, and pelvic organs. We spent most of the time in the office providing treatments for incontinence, erectile dysfunction, and related matters.

Clinic time also allowed for office-based surgeries like adult circumcision and vasectomy. Since I had been doing vasectomies as a student for two years, this was a time to hone an existing skill.

The urology surgeons had a different method, and I was not a big fan of it. They would place the patient in a reclining exam table used for women when doing pap smears. They would have the patient put his legs in the metal stirrups. This allows the testicle sac to hang loosely in the wind. The surgeon would sit on a stool facing the patient who could watch if he wanted.

One unfortunate (for some) staffing issue arose with the nurse that assisted these procedures. She was young, blond, and gorgeous. She would come into the room before the physician, to wash and prep the surgical area with a Betadine antibiotic solution. I would watch the poor, embarrassed face of the patient, as he dealt with it.

"Oh, come on now. Really?" the captive patients would comment, as the nurse entered and announced the plan.

Watching this always made me smile.

It was my day to do all the scheduled vasectomies. There were four scheduled one hour apart. We always offered the patient a Valium tablet to relax both him and the cremasteric muscle that could involuntarily pull the testicle up when cold or touched.

My first procedure finished early, and as I thought about the next one, it occurred to me that I was getting good at this procedure.

"The patient is prepped and ready, Doctor," said the attractive nurse from behind the cracked-open office door.

I walked briskly into the room, shook his hand, and said *hello* to my patient. He was a bit uncomfortable with a bright light shining on his groin covered with a sterile blue towel.

"What's the record for the fastest vasectomy done by your urology surgeons?" I asked the nurse.

"Fourteen minutes, sir," smiled the nurse. The patient was paying close attention now.

"Well then, today, we will beat that record," I responded, looking at the large military clock on the wall.

"No, no, really Doc," pleaded the patient. "Take your time, sir. Take your time."

We were done in eleven minutes flat.

Chapter 31 — Eczema

A 9-month-old African American baby I was examining was covered head-to-toe with a dry, scaly rash. He was crying. There were cracks in his skin that oozed a clear sticky liquid. Even his penis was involved. The palms of his hands and the soles of his feet were normal. He was the third child I had seen like this in a month on the pediatric rotation. This was the worst, and I did not understand what was causing it. All I could recommend was moisturizing lotions and rare use of steroid creams for bad areas.

What exactly is eczema? I asked myself again. My pediatric dermatology book noted 'it is a descriptive term used mistakenly as a diagnosis. It is a term used when a provider does not know what is causing a rash. The rash called eczema is dry, scaly, and itchy.' Often, it's all over the body. Vitamin D seems to help. If it were a fungal rash, it would be called tinea. Poison ivy and certain plants can cause a contact dermatitis that can mimic eczema.

I went in search of the attending pediatric physician. That day I got lucky, because she was African American and knew how to help.

"Severe eczema is more common in dark-skinned races," she explained in a whispered voice.

She motioned for me to move out of the hallway into a vacant exam room and continued in a soft voice.

"If you ask the mom when the rash started, you will discover it began right after she stopped breastfeeding. You will also find that the child is on a milk-based formula. He's allergic to the protein in the milk," she concluded.

"Why are we whispering?" I queried.

"Milk is an all-American food. The government subsidizes the industry. Studies proving the strong connection between milk and allergic reactions like eczema are primarily done in Europe. The milk industry can sue you if you imply milk can be bad for your health," she lectured.

"Even in pediatrics there's a reluctance to address the link between milk and problems in the darker-skinned races. Lactose (milk sugar) intolerance is common and causes bloating, abdominal pain, and foul-smelling farts across multiple races. But the eczema and milk connection is often scoffed at," she continued.

"Lactose intolerance is caused by the lack of the lactase enzyme needed to digest milk sugars, as you recall. Eczema is a real allergic reaction to the protein in milk. Over half the world's population avoids milk. Our patients with African or Eskimo ancestors come from countries where cow milk was never used for food. The result is, genetically, they have no ability to completely digest this food source."

I was amazed.

"What can I do for this boy?" I pleaded.

She smiled. "Actually, it's pretty simple. Educate the mom about it and get her to switch to a soy-based formula. Soy protein can also cause a mild reaction in these kids, but that is less common. I like to tell mothers that cow's milk is healthy for baby cows, but not for people."

"What about adding vitamin D since that's in cow milk, and it's supposed to help eczema?"

"That's an interesting point. Vitamin D was added to cow's milk in the 1930s because of an epidemic of rickets disease in children. Kids were working in factories back then, and Boston, for example, had eighty percent of the kids with rickets. The Pacific Northwest, where the sun seldom shines, had the problem from infancy to adult. Rickets causes soft bones and bowlegged kids. The lack of vitamin D prevents needed calcium absorption, so the government decided milk needed vitamin D for babies. The problem with that is fifty percent of the world population can't drink milk for reasons like eczema and lactose intolerance," she lectured softly.

"So, should I give this baby vitamin D, or is there enough in soymilk?" I whispered.

"The relatively new treatment plans for eczema do recommend adding vitamin D. It should help speed the healing process, but strict avoidance of milk and milk products like cheese is needed as the baby grows up. We have begun giving vitamin D to all newborn babies before we send them home. The whole world today hides from the sun, so even the moms are deficient."

Three months later, the baby came back for his one-year checkup, and his eczema was gone. Mom was thrilled. I was her hero. *Fun.*

Years later, at Fort Bragg, NC, where I worked in a clinic as a family physician, a mother brought her six-year-old son to me. The family had returned from a three-year assignment to Panama. The doctors there had been treating her son's severe case of 'eczema' for eighteen months with no improvement. The child scratched constantly and could not sleep. All the creams and lotions, mineral baths, and anti-fungal medications had failed to help.

I was one more stop in their quest for help. The child was miserable.

"Hello, young man," I started. His entire exposed skin area grabbed my attention. It was horrible. He had bumps and scratches and scars on his hands, arms, legs, and neck. His face was OK, but the neck along the hairline was red and raw from scratching. A clear yellow crust showed in areas where an infection was beginning.

I shook his hand and held it. He watched me curiously.

"Do your fingers itch too? Can I look at them for a minute?"

"Yes," he nodded.

There were cracks and faint skin burrows between his fingers in the web space. There were also a fair number of small red papules that were suspiciously like bug bites.

I learned about their medical battle to date, with multiple providers, and shook my head in disgust. It was a straightforward condition that was easy to recognize and cure.

He had scabies. These scabies mites burrow under the skin and lay their eggs there. Then they poop in their nest, tire of living there and move on to another place to burrow. *Yuk.*

"The good news is that we can help him quickly," I stated confidently to the mother. "I'm going to prescribe a cream for you to apply to his entire body tonight, from his ears to his toes. Do this at bedtime and wash it off in the morning. Do the same process again in one week to make sure. Wash the sheets in the morning in hot water both times. He has tiny bugs in his skin, and the lotion will kill them. He'll feel better in the morning. The rash will take a couple of weeks to heal back to normal."

"Bring him back to me, please, in three or four weeks so I can confirm we got it all. Sometimes, we need to retreat it," I finished, smiling.

The doubtful but hopeful mom took the written prescription, looked at it cautiously, and thanked me with a hint of hope in her voice.

Three weeks later, I saw, through the clinic glass door, the mother and her son coming up the walk. The boy was in the lead and was intent. I walked to the door and opened it.

The arms of a happy little child engulfed me. He would not let go.

"Thank you, thank you," he repeated over and over. His rash was gone. It was a good day.

The mother waited until he let go, wrapped her arms around me and whispered, "Thank you, Doctor. You are our savior."

One year later, I transferred to a new job. I was in the enviable position of Command Surgeon for the famous Army DELTA Force. A clinic medic told me that a soldier's wife was coming to see me for her eczema. He knew eczema was an interest of mine. She was a teacher and a professional soccer player. Her husband was a bit of a unit legend, and the medic made sure I knew.

The command had been involved in numerous stressful combat events. Her husband had survived with honor and military recognition, but he had also seen death up close and personal.

"I see why you were sent to me," I started as I closed the clinic room door and held out my hand. She shook it and nodded. Her entire visible body was covered in a rash. Even her face was involved, and that was unusual for most eczema type rashes.

We moved to an exam room. "Let me look at all of you. You have your bra on, so just lift your shirt so I can see the abdomen, chest, and back."

The rash was severe and everywhere — except for one area. Her back was clear in a large, oval, mid-back area. Medically speaking, that ruled out a common cause because those would also involve the back.

I knew what it was, and creams would not help. "Tell me a bit about your work and soccer successes or challenges," I requested casually.

After a long, detailed list of all the stresses in her life, including wondering when her husband would disappear again on another mission, she paused.

"I think I can help you. The itching is causing you to scratch all over, and your fingernails are causing most of the damage," I began. She nodded with interest.

"I will give you an 'anti-itch' pill that I want you to take at night. It won't work immediately. As a matter of fact, in the first five days, you're going to start thinking, 'That damn doc doesn't know anything.' But, in the following week, you're going to wake up and realize you slept better, and the itch is better. I will want to see you back here in one month. By then, we will know if the medicine is working as planned." I smiled and hoped she would not challenge me further.

The pill I gave her was an anti-depressant. She would look that up, of course, and know it when I saw her next time, so I added, "This pill falls into the category of an anti-anxiety medicine, but we use it for itching too." I was not lying, but I did stretch the truth a bit.

One month later, she returned as planned and presented me with her skin clear of all disease. Her rash was gone. It had been self-inflicted. I realized that when I observed the only clear skin area was where her fingernails could not reach.

A treatment bonus event occurred a few months later. Her husband walked by my office, looking in as he passed. Then he did that two more times.

"Sergeant, did you want to talk to me?" I inquired, pretty sure that he did.

He would not come in the room, but he peeked around the doorjamb and began, "Sir. What you did for my wife......can you do that for me?"

"Come in, please, and we can talk about that."

Post-Traumatic Stress Disorder (PTSD) is impossible to avoid in war. This amazing warrior had done it all and had used his superb skills to save lives in a real hellhole. He had lost friends and seen fellow warriors die. His coping mechanism was similar to his wife's. They both chose to push themselves to their physical limits. It did not work. Their brains had abnormal hormone activity caused by stresses in their lives. Even his teammates knew that he was pushing too hard. Yes, he won physical contests, but he did not sleep, and he did not go home when he could. He worked out day and night.

"Sergeant, I'll give you the same medicine that I gave your wife. It helped her, and it will help you," I concluded after careful exploration of his concerns.

I started him on the same anti-depressant that had helped his wife. With treatment, he could control the PTSD symptoms that all combat veterans must deal with. It helped. It thrilled me later to learn that he had left the unit, made Sergeant Major, and was enjoying a healthy life with a normal wife.

Chapter 32 – Don't Operate – Surgery

General surgery was a grueling rotation. A call from the emergency room was often something terrible. Appendicitis, diverticulitis with perforation, bowel cancers, thrombosed hemorrhoids, and knife or bullet wounds presented at every hour of the day or night. Being on call at night was exhausting. Surgeons were often reported as the specialty that 'ate its young.'

"A chance to cut is a chance to cure."

"A day off means missed surgeries."

As residents, we oversaw the recovery ward and the hospital ward where patients were being managed before and after surgery. Wounds needed care, central IV lines needed placement, ultrasounds, biopsies, and more took up much of the day and night. The emergency room would call, and tasks were redistributed, while we went to see what had walked in the door.

"I can't stand the pains in my stomach anymore," she sobbed in distress.

We admitted her. The next day I was at her bedside. The morning rounds were done, and she was scheduled for surgery that morning. The plan was to do exploratory surgery to look for anything to explain her daily and constant, severe pain. She had no fevers.

Her labs were all normal, and the CT (computerized tomography) scan of her abdomen only showed a non-specific bowel gas pattern. The tears in her eyes were real, and her exam always elicited pain when tapping or poking on her abdomen. Unexpectedly, we could not find a specific focus of her pain. The gallbladder typically hurt in the right upper quadrant. The ovaries always hurt low down on a pelvic exam. Bowel perforations were more common in the left lower quadrant and came with a fever. Her pain seemed to be everywhere. It did not fit into a neat little diagnostic box.

I had a few minutes before I had to be elsewhere, so I did what family physicians do. I talked to her. She came from Thailand, and her entire family was there. She had come to the U.S. married to an enlisted man she had met in Thailand. Her family was happy for her. The land of plenty awaited her.

They had one child - a two-year-old girl but had hoped for a boy. Her husband was assigned to a transportation company that supported the

82nd Airborne. Her English was fair but heavily accented. I thought she was probably pretty once, but now her face and eyes just showed pain.

I went to the operating room for the first surgery of the afternoon dressed in fresh green scrubs. Paper disposable slippers covered my shoes. My job was to hold retractors, snip sutures, and dab or suction blood. It was fun looking inside a body to see actual living organs in action. Today, however, I was bothered by our next scheduled surgery patient from Thailand.

"John, I need to share a concern with you about our next patient," I stated while we were waiting for the anesthesiologist to join us. I was speaking to the senior surgical resident in the pre-op area where we washed our hands.

"Go ahead, please. It is a confusing presentation."

"I talked to her after rounds and picked up on some disturbing issues. Her family is all in Thailand. Finances are not good, and she has a two-year-old daughter they had hoped would be a boy. Her husband is an enlisted man with a boring job," I started.

"We see a fair number of Asian women married to junior enlisted men in our clinic. One of the common complaints that I get from these ladies is abdominal pain. When we have time to talk to them alone, we see they're unhappy, and usually in an abusive relationship," I observed.

"We label it as irritable bowel syndrome. When I see that, I treat it with antidepressants. That is usually effective. When it doesn't help, I often learn about a husband that physically or mentally abuses his spouse. I think your next exploratory surgery is a case like that," I concluded.

"I did not want to cut her open," John stated. "It seemed like we had to find something given the nature of her pains. Why don't you get a social work consult started, and we can postpone her surgery until we have a better reason," he said gratefully.

I hoped I was right because it would save her unnecessary surgery. I wished I was wrong because there was little a doctor could do to help her home situation or abuse.

I learned from the social worker that I was correct.

Chapter 33 - The Amazing Thyroid

The thyroid is a silent friend and a miserable enemy. It can poop-out partially or entirely. It lives in the front of the neck and can grow to enormous sizes and is called a goiter when it enlarges. Queen Elizabeth I, of England, was rumored to have a large visible goiter, so she invented the royal clothing style with a large paper collar to wear. It would have hidden her goiter.

It can explode into overactivity. Hyperthyroid is an overactive thyroid condition. A thyroid cancer nodule can cause it, but commonly the gland is overstimulated by an autoimmune response following a simple cold virus infection.

There are areas in the country where new thyroid disease is essentially unheard of, and regions (like the South) where it is common. The temperatures in these Southern states are more conducive to certain viruses' reproduction and growth. One theory that is gaining credence with DNA technology is that the Coxsackievirus and Echovirus are both responsible for thyroid diseases.

"You will have to admit this patient to the wards," came the plea from the emergency room doctor on the phone. "We don't know what's wrong with her, but she can't go home."

I was the resident in charge of the inpatient ward. We were busy, but I went to the ER to see this mystery patient.

"She has been having increasing bouts of disorientation at home," began the ER doc. "Her family says she can't remember their names or even what a saltshaker is used for. She has no stroke symptoms, and her voice is normal but a bit slow. We did a CT scan and a bunch of labs, and they're all normal. You need to take her upstairs and figure out what's wrong, please," he pleaded.

"Let me take a look," I nodded and moved to her exam room.

I pulled the curtain back to reveal a woman in her sixties, covered with a sheet. The first thing I noticed was a large pale scar on her neck, so I started there.

"When did she have her thyroid surgery?" I asked her son, standing nearby.

"Oh, that was at least thirty years ago when she lived in Mexico," he answered thoughtfully.

"Is she taking her thyroid medicine?" I continued as the logical next step in the exam process.

"No, she has never taken any medications, except a vitamin pill sometimes. She hates medicines," he responded.

I considered that a minute. If she had her thyroid removed over thirty years ago and never took thyroid replacements, she would be severely hypothyroid. It is a rare condition I have read about but never seen.

"Is her face rounder than it used to be?" I started. Her eyes got big, and she started shaking her head *yes*, with her hands making a gesture of roundness around her face. 'Moon face' is a physical finding of severe long-standing hypothyroidism. The head will appear to be rounder than years before, and old pictures can show a noticeable difference.

"Does she have dry skin?" I asked next, and she kicked off the sheet, nodding again.

Her skin resembled that of an alligator. It looked and felt hard, dry and cracked. It stunned me. I did not need to ask the rest of the questions that would confirm what I already knew, so I excused myself and found the ER doctor.

"You might want to look at her skin, face, and neck. You will note a thyroid surgery scar and discover that she hasn't had thyroid replacement medications for over thirty years. This is a very cool case. You need to order a TSH blood test and likely start her on thyroid medications. Hypothyroidism explains all of her symptoms." He was stunned.

"My work here is done," I declared smugly as I waved over my shoulder, walking away. "Gotta get back to the wards," I smiled, and walked away with an impudent and unappreciated swagger. This time I got it right – not always so in the coming months of learning.

The next month included full days in the clinic. I would see ten patients in the morning and ten in the afternoon. It was late in the afternoon when I met an eighty-two-year-old lady with shortness of breath.

"I have not been able to catch my breath for the last few months, and it has gotten worse this week," she started.

"I have felt like I had a fever with hot, sweaty skin, but my temperature is normal. My heart is beating in my chest, and I can't seem to breathe right," she finished.

The exam revealed a heart rate of 120 beats per minute, warm moist skin, and lungs with crackling sounds at the bases of both lungs. These are the sounds associated with congestive heart failure (CHF).

"Do you use salt with iodine in it? Or do you use sea salt?" I asked, thinking about her thyroid function.

"I use Morton salt which has iodine in it, I think. Why do you ask?"

"There's an interesting bit of history related to iodine and salt. Back in the frontier days, before refrigeration, our settlers in the Midwest started getting goiters and thyroid problems. Iodine is in seafood, and transport to the Midwest was impossible. Once the government figured out that the cause of thyroid disease in our settlers was due to iodine deficiency, they looked for a food to put iodine in. The Mormons had the Great Salt Lake, lots of goiters, and no seafood. So, iodine was put in everyone's salt," I lectured.

"Well, that isn't me. I eat fish every week and use regular salt."

"OK," I nodded. "Let's get an EKG of her heart and a chest X-ray of her lungs," I said to the nurse. "I don't like the sound of her lungs or heart. After that, send her to the lab for blood work," I directed.

I thought about what I should order because I was confused as to what caused her distress, so I ordered all the standard stuff, looking for infection or heart failure. I added a thyroid test just in case.

When she returned, I had the X-ray and EKG results, but the labs would not be available until the next day. The X-ray confirmed my CHF suspicions.

"I'm going to start you on a beta-blocker to slow down your heart and a water pill to help you pee out fluid in your lungs and help you breathe better," I explained. "I will want you to come back next week, but in the meantime, I'm putting in a consult to the cardiologists to see if they have any other concerns or suggestions," I finished.

The next day I started, as usual, looking at the previous day's labs. The thyroid lab from my eighty-two-year-old lady was grossly abnormal. It showed her thyroid was extraordinarily overactive and was producing lots of excess thyroid hormone. This would explain all her symptoms. With excess thyroid hormone production, the heart will go into overdrive, and the heart rate will increase dramatically. The body temperature will elevate, and metabolic rates in cells and organs will increase. If not treated, it can be fatal.

I called her. "Can you please come back to see me today? Your labs came back with one important abnormality. Your thyroid is overactive, and that is affecting your heart. Do you feel any better on the new medicines?" I asked.

She did feel stronger, so an ultrasound was ordered ASAP. It identified an abnormal solid spot. A nuclear iodine thyroid uptake scan followed the next day. It showed that an area, in the left lobe, was overactive and suspicious for thyroid cancer.

The next week, a surgeon removed the left lobe of her thyroid gland. He preserved the four small parathyroid glands which are embedded in the surrounding thyroid tissue. These glands have a different function, are necessary for calcium management, and were operating fine. The next month she returned for her post-operative checkup.

"I feel like a new woman," she exclaimed, smiling.

"It is more important to know what sort of patient has a disease, than what disease a patient has."
William Ostler

NEW ATTENDING PHYSICIAN

Chapter 34 – On my Own

I completed my three-year residency training in June. I was an MD, but no longer under supervision. We traveled across the country again and moved the family to Fort Bragg, NC. In August, I reported for duty.

I dressed proudly and meticulously for my first day as an attending physician at Womack Army Medical Center. I was part of the teaching staff that would oversee one of the best Family Medicine residency programs in the military. My uniform was fresh and pressed, and I decided to wear my ribbons, Army parachute wings, and Navy SEAL insignia over the left breast pocket. Uniform regulations allowed other service qualification badges to be worn. It was a statement to the new staff that I had been blessed with prior service. It would affect how they managed my indoctrination.

My three years in residency had taught me enough about the Army that I was comfortable with the rank and the relatively new uniform. Eighteen years in the Navy still found me using words like *bulkhead* for a wall, *ladder* for stairs, and *head* for bathroom or latrine. It made for confused Army responses. These Navy words were unknown to most soldiers.

I reported to Major John Johnson, the Residency Director, as part of my check-in.

"Welcome to Womack, Bob," he began while shaking my hand. "We're short doctors during this summer transition and new-resident orientation time. We were expecting you today, and since this week is an orientation week, you are assigned to the labor deck tonight on call. Can you handle that?" he queried.

"Yes, sir. That will be fine," I said with anticipation and feeling quite comfortable with obstetrics after three years in residency, where I had been on the labor deck often with my patients. This would be fun.

At 5 PM, I showed up on the labor deck and informed the front desk I was the new Family physician, and they gave me a tour of the modern, fully equipped floor. They directed me to the locker area and physician break and sleep area where I changed into scrubs, from the large pile of green scrubs positioned in the locker room. After slipping into my starched, long white coat with my name embroidered over the pocket, I sauntered out to the nurse's station.

"Welcome, Doctor Adams," began the head nurse.

"We have eight beds in active labor now, but none are close to delivery. Your resident tonight is Doctor Daphne Jones. She'll be here soon after the inpatient team finishes checking out the ward patients to her. There's a nurse-midwife managing her patient in Room 1. You might want to run to the cafeteria and get dinner soon. It looks like we might have a busy night," she finished, smiling. It was an old-hat routine for her. The doctors and residents came and went. Her job, in part, was to keep us oriented and safe.

After a quick meal in the basement cafeteria I returned to the deck with a new spring in my step. I was the real thing now – a doctor with eight new lives in my future.

The sun set, and a full moon rose. We knew the labor deck could get crazy on the night of a full moon. The moon affects the ocean tides, and it seemed to pull on the amniotic fluid inside a pregnant woman's uterus just as effectively. Emergency rooms report more shootings and violent assaults on the night of a full moon.

"Hey, look at Room 5," I stated with concern. I had been leaning on the nurse station counter and chatting with the grey-haired head nurse. There were twelve labor monitors on the wall behind her. Eight of them were in constant motion displaying contraction strength, frequency, vitals, and fetal heart rate. The fetal heart rate in Room 5 was dropping precipitously in a bad way. It was a sign of fetal distress and needed rapid intervention.

"Damn," I said to the nurse, now looking over her shoulder at the monitor. "Who's the attending physician tonight?"

"Um, that would be you, sir," she pronounced.

"Whoops. Well, damn. Come with me, please," I whispered as I moved adroitly to the room in question.

"Hi, I'm Doctor Adams," I stated as I moved bedside. "Roll over onto your hands and knees, please," I directed as the nurse positioned herself to handle the IV line, monitor wires, and bedding.

"Your baby is showing some signs of distress, so I'm going to reach in and push the baby's head back up a bit," I began, in as calm a voice as I could muster.

She rolled over, took the pillow the nurse handed her and moved her buttocks back toward me. There was leaking amniotic fluid, and it looked stained, like the baby may have had a bowel movement. This added an additional risk factor to the pending delivery.

"Quick, give me the…. the…." I could not remember the name of the medicine I wanted.

"Give me the contraction-go-away medicine," I finished urgently.

"Terbutaline?" smiled the nurse, who was enjoying the moment.

"Yes, please. Give one mg now," I panted, remembering the protocol.

"Do you want that IM or IV?" asked the nurse, still having fun at my expense.

I had my hand inside the soon-to-be-mothers vaginal opening holding upward pressure on the presenting head.

"Dang, I don't know. What do you normally do?" I asked exasperated.

"IV usually," she smiled.

"Yes, please. Do that now, IV."

She already had the syringe in hand and injected it into the intravenous line port. We both watched the monitor as the contractions lessened and stopped. The magic of modern medicine made me smile.

The baby's heart rate returned to a regular resting pattern, and we rolled our patient onto her back again. The nurse and I breathed a sigh of relief.

"Please stay here with her," I directed. "I'm going to find our obstetrician and let her know we may have a C-section in her future." The nurse smiled and nodded. I listened to her soothing the worried patient as I fast-walked to the physician call room in search of the on-call obstetrician able to assist with the C-section if needed.

The night passed in a blur. We had three more labor admissions, and we delivered five. Our lady in Room 5 had an uneventful vaginal delivery of a seven-pound two-ounce baby girl with a full head of black hair.

The military C-section rate is much lower than the civilian rate. This is because of malpractice threats that plague obstetricians daily. Obstetrics has been one of the most sued specialties. The logic was simple and sad. If the baby showed any sign of distress (which is common temporarily), and you allowed a vaginal delivery, then any adverse outcome is inviting a lawsuit. But, if you did a C-section, the argument would be that 'we did all we could.'

My C-section rate was about five percent of the women I managed and delivered. The civilian rate is about thirty-two percent. The C-section rate on a Friday is higher than the other days of the week. Doctors often promote C-sections on Friday to avoid weekend deliveries.

It was a great first night as a full-fledged, on-my-own attending physician.

Chapter 35 - Invade Haiti (Almost) – Keep Me Alive

After arriving at Fort Bragg, NC, I was invited to recertify in static line parachuting so I could be assigned to the 82nd Airborne Division if it went to war. There were ten other jump qualified doctors, but they would need more if they got the call to go somewhere 'hot.' This division was America's ready force, able to be airborne in 48 hours.

I had not jumped from an airplane in seven years during medical school and residency. I had tried to but was informed it was against regulations for doctors in residency training.

My first refresher jump at Fort Bragg, wearing my new Army uniform, was easy and fun. I had been jumping static line and freefall for many years and had served on the freefall parachute team that traveled the U.S. doing jump demonstrations. This was a reminder of why I liked my job in the military, and it came with extra jump pay to boot.

September arrived with a bombshell. The family was settled into our new house, and I had made one freefall jump with SEALs in the area to recertify in freefall parachuting. Life was calm and enjoyable.

"Sir, this is the Womack Staff Duty Officer. You are released from your current duties and assigned to the 82nd Airborne, 2nd of the 325 Air Infantry Regiment, effective immediately. Please report to their command headquarters as soon as you can. They're expecting you," ordered the voice on the phone.

After a brief discussion, with me trying to find out more, all I could discover was they needed me there now. They instructed me not to call home until briefed at the new unit.

This was an unexpected development for a new physician learning how the Army worked, but I knew what it meant. The Division was going operational.

The hours that followed found me in a briefing announcing an invasion of Haiti. Operation Uphold Democracy would begin in 48 hours. They planned a 3,500-man parachute assault onto the island of Haiti.

I went home that evening and began packing my gear for a combat parachute invasion of another country. We would all report back in the morning to begin a lock-down phase to prepare for the assault. Phone lines were blocked, and military police guarded roads in and out of the Division area. No one was to come or go.

At the first sand-table briefing, I learned that they had assigned me to jump from aircraft number one. I was tasked to jump in with the unit commander. They would place me in the middle of the jumper line so that if we jumped too early or too late, I would more likely end up where I was needed. The others might find themselves on rooftops, as the time over the drop zone was short.

"Sir, I understand you requested me to be on your aircraft because you liked the fact that I was a SEAL and more senior than the other docs. I need to tell you that I have no Army operational experience and don't know what I'm supposed to do once we hit the ground."

"Doc, listen. All I need you to do is keep me alive if something happens to me," he stated commandingly.

"Yes, sir. I can do that," I responded, with false confidence.

The story of 3,500 paratroopers launching in the night to fly four hours to Haiti and take the island by force was suppressed. My wife later reported the local news had done a live broadcast of sixty-four large aircraft taking off from the local air force base that evening.

She observed that the entire town was aware that all the military surplus stores had stayed open all night the previous night selling war-related materials. The entire stock of summer field uniforms had been withdrawn from the dry cleaners in town. The knife store in the post exchange set up a table outside with a large sign 'free knife sharpening.' There was a long line. The secret was the community's to keep, but Fort Bragg had seen and done this before.

Two hours after the launch, the acting president of Haiti surrendered. General Colin Powell had informed him the entire division was two hours out. The sixty-four aircraft were turned around and brought back. We were tired and wet from loading in the rain, but we had won a war without firing a shot.

Chapter 36 – Tongue Lesion – Call the Code

She was thirty-one years old, a mother of two small children, and had never smoked a cigarette. She had come to ask about her tongue. There was a white spot on the side of her tongue that would not go away. It had been there for over two weeks. I examined it with my light, and it appeared smooth and somewhat solid. It was not a fungus or a sore. The rest of her mouth and neck exams were normal, but the lesion needed to be biopsied.

I called my favorite ENT surgeon on his cell phone, and he agreed to see her that afternoon.

"I will be honest with you," I told her. "I don't think this is something bad, but we need to make sure. It could be a type of oral wart or other inflammatory tissue. Don't worry about it until we tell you to worry," I smiled confidently.

She thanked me, made a note of where the ENT clinic was, and left. Her medical history was reassuring. She was young, attractive, healthy, and ate a healthy diet. I scribbled a note in her chart, placed it in the outbox, and moved to my next patient.

The next day, my phone rang. It was the ENT surgeon.

"What's up, Mike?" I started.

"Bob, I got the biopsy back, and the news isn't good. Your lady has a spindle cell tumor of her tongue."

"What the heck is that?" I stuttered.

He explained that it was a rare form of cancer that was dangerous and often aggressive. The tongue was an unusual place for it to occur. He asked if I wanted to tell her, or if he should. Since I knew nothing about it or the treatment options, I requested that he call her.

"I plan to do a complete surgical excision right away," he went on. "I'll get an MRI of the head and neck, as this tumor is more common in the neck areas, and I'll copy you on the results and treatment plan," he finished.

I called her later to see if she had any questions after I did some research of my own. As always, I was upbeat and positive. We beat cancer often. She was young and healthy.

"We can beat this."

The MRI came back, noting the possible involvement of one or two neck lymph nodes. The tongue surgical excision pathology came back 'margins clear.' That meant that the surgeon had removed the entire tongue tumor, but the involved lymph nodes added additional concern. If the tumor cells had moved into the lymph system, her battle would be more complicated.

Two weeks later, I was invited to assist in an exploratory neck surgery to remove the lymph nodes, now proven positive for metastatic cancer. The patient wanted me there. As her family doctor, I took care of her husband and two children also.

My job consisted of holding the retractors and keeping the tissue dry by dabbing or holding pressure on bleeding areas while the surgeon tied off and removed the abnormal tissues.

He cut a large flap of neck skin in an L-shape and began to peel it back from the muscles underneath. It was about four inches in length and three inches along the bottom edge, so we could fold back the skin revealing the vessels and soft tissue of the neck.

I held the flap back and dabbed gently at a small area oozing blood. The surgeon was tying a suture at the base of an enlarged lymph node.

"Gentlemen," crooned the anesthesiologist at the head of the table, "whatever you're doing now, please stop immediately."

We both froze and looked at the monitors. Her heart rate slowed precipitously, and in a few seconds, we watched the monitor display a flat line. Her heart had stopped beating.

"Oh, oh, oh!" came the shocked reply from Mike. I waited for his next command, but when it did not come, I took charge.

I glanced in alarm at the OR tech. "Please lower the head of the bed. Lower the table to waist level and call a Code Blue to this room. Doctor Mansfield will begin chest compressions now."

Mike's eyes were wide with shock. He began chest compressions while the anesthesiologist announced he was administering IV drugs to stimulate the heart.

"Damn, this has never happened to me before," whispered Mike with surprise and panic in his voice as he pushed up and down firmly on her chest.

I watched the monitor and noted some new cardiac activity. "Stop compressions and check pulse, please," I directed, and Mike stopped. Sweat stained his paper surgical cap.

Mike palpated her wrist, and the anesthesiologist reached for her carotid artery on the non-surgical side. I could see the pulsatile movement in the exposed neck vessels.

"We have a pulse," remarked both doctors. The entire entourage breathed a sigh of relief. It appeared that pulling on the nerves in the neck had overstimulated the vagus nerve that ran alongside the carotid artery. These nerves conduct signals that control the heart rate. Overstimulation of them slows the heart rate. We had done that a bit too well.

The surgery continued, and we removed the offending tissue. I had to tell her husband in the waiting room about our bit of excitement. I told him her heart had stopped, but only for a brief period. We believed that the surgery went well despite the unexpected drama and added that I had seen this happen before in routine operations because of the strength of anesthesia. He appeared relieved.

We did not beat her cancer. Six months after the initial diagnosis, she died of cancer and its rapid progression.

I still endure a sense of loss and failure.

Chapter 37 - Levine's Sign Heart Attack

"Doctor, something's wrong," came the cry from the room behind me.

I looked through the doorway and saw an elderly lady in obvious distress.

"Here I come," I announced decisively with no idea what I would see. The morning had been routine. I was visiting the twelve patients on the inpatient service. It was a Saturday, and I was covering for the internal medicine team in the local community hospital. I was moonlighting to make extra money, and so they could have a day off.

I rushed into the room to find three family members looking at a thin, dark-skinned lady in obvious pain. Her left hand was clenched over her left chest, and her eyes were wide. Her mouth was open like she wanted to say something, but no sound emerged. It was the first time I had ever witnessed Levine's sign.

Doctor Levine was a cardiologist who earned notoriety decades ago by describing the clenched fist over the heart that I was witnessing. All doctors learn that it usually means a patient is having cardiac chest pain.

I remembered this lady from an hour before when I had rounded on her. *Rounding* is the term we used describing the process of visiting our patients and reviewing their charts and writing necessary orders for the nurses to implement. She had been moved to the internal medicine Step-down Ward from the Cardiac Intensive Care Unit after admission for a heart attack. She was a 'no-code' patient who had signed a DNR (Do Not Resuscitate) request.

"OK, gang - it seems like Mom is having another heart attack," I stated softly.

"She has made it clear that she does not want us to shock her or take any painful or heroic measures in this situation, so I will give her morphine to ease the pain." The family all nodded.

"Nurse, please get me ten milligrams of morphine to give IV, STAT," I requested to the duty nurse standing at the door. She had heard the family call. STAT is a term derived from the Latin word 'statum,' which means 'immediately.' It implies an urgency that all medical personnel recognize.

"Mrs. Mullen, it looks like you are having another heart attack, so I'll give you some medicine to make the pain go away," I announced. Her head bobbed in understanding.

The medicine arrived in less than a minute, and the nurse grabbed the IV line, showed me the vial, saw me nod, and turned the drip rate to full flow. She pushed the morphine steadily into the IV line, and in a few seconds, we could see the benefit. Mrs. Mullen's face lost the expression of pain, and she relaxed.

I held her right hand, where the IV line was, and a daughter held her other hand. My mind rushed, as I tried to think of other things I might do. Her DNR request legally required me to avoid causing pain by shocking her heart, intubating her, or doing chest compressions. I could order an EKG to confirm what I already knew. Her medications included a nitroglycerine patch for twelve hours a day. Her patch was visible on the arm I held. More nitroglycerine would not help.

I chose to wait and see.

Since 1912 physicians have used morphine to ease the pain of a heart attack or angina pain. It was then thought to dilate heart vessels and help prevent heart muscle damage. In reality, it slightly increases the risk of dying from certain types of heart attacks.

The calmness in the room increased as the morphine took effect. The family and the nurse watched with me. I reached for the patient's wrist to feel her pulse. I did this for my benefit and for the watchful and confused family.

Her death came soundlessly and not unexpectedly. Her mouth opened slowly, and her eyes rolled up. There were a few reflex breaths triggered by the brainstem responding to the lack of oxygen. Then chest movement stopped. The pulse stopped, so I put on my stethoscope and listened in three places for her heartbeat. I knew that I would not hear it, but it was necessary for what I would be required to do. I needed to certify the time of death.

Her eyes were closed, and the room remained silent except for her daughter's soft sobs.

I glanced at the clock on the wall. "Time of death 9:23 AM," I stated to the nurse who nodded.

"I am so sorry for your loss, and I'm certain that with the medicine, she did not have pain with her passing. Is there anything I can do for you all?"

The nurse took over and ushered me out of the room to give the family time to mourn. She knew what to do and how to do it. The room would be empty and clean soon.

There is an almost magical calm that comes with death. All experience it, and it is always moving. The delivery of a child and the death of a loved one are events that physicians are blessed to experience. Life is different after such events. For me, it reinforces that there is a soul, and life comes and goes with a reverence that is impossible to describe.

Chapter 38 – Tobacco and Death

"You're nineteen years old and twenty-four weeks pregnant. This is your family's first child. You need to quit smoking. You're harming your unborn child," I observed as passionately as I could.

She burst into tears. "Doctor Adams, I can't quit. I've tried and tried. I just can't do it. It's impossible. Can you help me? I know I'm hurting my baby. Please?" she sobbed.

"There are medicines that we use to help tobacco addiction," I began. "But, unfortunately, they're not safe in pregnancy. You'll have to do this on your own. I know you can do it. Keep thinking about your child. Remember the money you'll save. Lots of good things will happen. Your taste will come back. Your clothes and car will smell good again. You'll be so proud of yourself," I exclaimed in my best cheerleader voice.

I repeated this encouragement each time she came in. At thirty-six weeks gestation, I began seeing her weekly. The pregnancy was progressing as expected, and at each visit, she again committed to quitting.

As a family physician, I enjoy the privilege of delivering a woman's child and caring for the newborn as it grows up. 'Womb to tomb care.'

Two weeks after her delivery, she stopped by my office. She was doing well, breastfeeding her newborn, and still smoking.

"Doctor Adams look," she said, unwrapping the blanket from the pretty little girl in her arms.

"Isn't she beautiful? And look, there's nothing wrong with her," she stated with relief and pride.

"She is beautiful," I responded. Her delivery, at full term, had gone well. She had pushed for two hours and delivered her daughter without needing an episiotomy. All-natural. The child weighed 5 pounds, 9 ounces.

I wanted to tell her the child was smaller than it should be. Her smoking had caused this. Her child might have respiratory or developmental issues later in life.

Not today. The future was uncertain. She would quit one day.

"I'm thrilled for you both," I smiled as I hugged them both.

I saw another pregnant lady later that week. She was taking her prenatal vitamins, and her weight was appropriate.

I began my standard dialog to help her quit. Studies reported that there was a twenty-five percent success rate when a doctor merely encouraged their patient to stop. I would keep trying.

"Don't you read the side of your cigarette packages?" I continued. "It says on the pack that smoking may cause harm to your unborn child."

"Yes, I know. But I don't smoke *those* cigarettes," she concluded truthfully.

I had no response as I stared at her with my wide eyes blinking.

My father knew he would die young and told me so before he died. It was a choice. He asked me to understand that he had no regrets. He had lived a good life and watched his three children grow into adulthood.

He would leave our mother too soon, and hold my son, who was named after him, just once.

Over the years, I have tried my best to assist patients with quitting, and most do eventually stop. Life, family, and medical issues impact their willpower.

"Let's see now," I often say. "You have maybe six years to live," I continue at the end of a typical office visit conversation.

"You should plan to die at sixty-three-years-old as my dad did. The good news is, you won't have to worry about retirement or Medicare, which starts at age sixty-five. Also, make sure you sign up for early social security benefits at age sixty-two. After all these years paying into it, at least you can get one year of benefits," I say sincerely and sarcastically.

"OK, Doc. Yeah, sure. I really am trying to quit," they would typically state and smile uncertainly. I shake their hands tightly as they leave to remind them that we are a team.

That conversation is part of every day that I see patients. Smokers know it is killing them. Some hate it. Some can't imagine life without it.

One of my patients had prostate cancer at age fifty-three. His prostate had been surgically removed, and he had completed radiation treatments. I walked into the room, smiling with my hand out. The air reeked of his stale rancid breath, which made me almost gag. As is always the case with heavy smokers, they would finish a cigarette before walking in. If I ran late, they would slip outside to smoke another and rush back. We were not able to use the room again until it had been fumigated. They had no idea how bad they stunk. Food did not taste normal, and their smell was impaired. Sometimes the damage to these senses was permanent.

"You have to know that your smoking caused your cancer," I noted.

"Yes, I know. But, look, you need to understand something too. I started smoking at six years old. Dad gave me my first cigarette. I don't remember a day in my life that I did not smoke. It's the only life I know, and I can't even imagine life without a cigarette," he concluded miserably but sincerely.

I had no good response.

"You are likely to die sooner than you want," I tried on my next patient of the day. I was talking to a patient that I knew well and liked a lot. He had heard this all before.

"Doc, seriously," he began. "Everyone in my family smokes. All of us. And we all die in our sixties. I understand that, and I'm OK with that."

"The FDA makes sure my cigarettes are safe, don't they?" asked one lady later in the day. I had heard this question before.

"No, ma'am. The FDA and the government do not monitor tobacco product ingredients for safety. The industry works very hard to make cigarettes as consumable and as addictive as possible. They add some deadly poisonous ammonia to make the nicotine more addictive, and chemicals found in anti-freeze make it sweeter and more comfortable to inhale. Then you set these chemicals on fire and inhale them. They actually dissolve your lung tissue until you eventually need oxygen to breathe.

"Well, then I will need to quit. Can you please tell me when I am going to need oxygen? I'll plan to quit the day before," she said thoughtfully.

Once again, I was at a loss for words. It is a terrible addiction and one that doctors must fight daily across every specialty. Babies of smokers get more ear infections, their children start smoking more frequently, respiratory infections are more common, pregnancies miscarry, and adults die too young.

"Tobacco doesn't really cause cancer does it?" asked my close friend as he puffed on his cigarette during a visit to his house.

"I'll answer that question with a history lesson. There was essentially no lung cancer in the world until decades after World War I. I read an article by a physician that practiced in the 1930s, recalling his first case of lung cancer. It was so rare then that he called all the other doctors and students to come to see it. It was diagnosed in an ex-soldier from the past war." I began.

"Over the next few years, this doctor explained, he began seeing cases of lung cancer quite regularly, and they were mostly in ex-soldiers. Two interesting bits of history made this happen. First, the machine rolled cigarette was invented in 1880, and second, the American entry into World War I in 1917 found the American Red Cross and the German Army giving cartons of cigarettes to every deploying soldier. Germany recognized the link in 1929 and began its post-war tobacco fight. It took a few decades, but ever since the 1930s, lung cancer – caused by smoking – has become a daily battle for doctors around the world. So, you tell me, is this all coincidence, or is tobacco your enemy?" I finished.

Five years later, he was diagnosed with bladder cancer, which is most commonly caused by smoking.

Tobacco use is decreasing steadily in the United States. Education is working, but usage is increasing in lesser developed countries as businesses move their marketing overseas.

I will never run out of patients.

Chapter 39 – 24-Hour Hospital On-Call

I was in debt after graduation from my three years of residency training. We had two kids and a $50,000 loan to pay when I received the hoped-for orders to Fort Bragg, NC.

Before I arrived in North Carolina, I called ahead to the Cape Fear Hospital in downtown Fayetteville, NC, and asked if they needed any help. They said yes.

I began the paperwork with them right away and readied myself to take a weekend twenty-four-hour call to help the hospital. It involved taking calls for admissions from the emergency room, rounding on patients on the wards, and responding to codes in the Intensive Care Unit (ICU), Cardiac Care Unit (CCU), and Surgical Intensive Care Unit (SICU). My military training had prepared me well, and I wanted to get out of debt.

The extra pay was good, and the often-exhausting twenty-four-hour days were both exhilarating and frightening. I would see conditions that were rare in the military. Drug overdoses, marijuana-induced psychoses, dialysis patients in renal failure, and terminal illnesses were common challenges in a community hospital.

I saw the vast differences in care that occurred when money was a motivator. Money worked both ways. In one way, doctors were urged to generate as much income as possible by ordering multiple specialty consults, laboratory tests, X-rays, and advanced diagnostic studies. In another way, these same tests were ordered to document what was not there. We spent the insurance money on unnecessary tests to document that we did not miss something rare. Malpractice threats affected patient care decisions.

"Doctor Adams, this is the charge nurse today in the ER. Doctor Patel would like you to see a patient here with bilateral pneumonia and a white count of zero. He's a cancer patient."

"Oh, crap. You know he has no chance of survival without white blood cells?" I responded.

"Yes, sir, we know. But the family and the patient want everything possible done, so we would need you to admit him, please."

"Of course. I'll be right there," I concluded by phone. It was 10 PM on a Saturday, and I had finished in the SICU where an open-heart surgery patient needed evaluation. Orders had been written to deal with breathing issues and ventilator settings.

"Sir, I'm Doctor Adams," I began, now in the ER. "I'm sorry to tell you that your X-rays show that both your lungs are full of pneumonia and fluid. That's why your breathing is so difficult."

He watched me with bright, fearful eyes while he huffed and puffed in the oxygen mask. He nodded. His wife was bedside and holding his hand.

"Unfortunately, there's a bigger problem. Your chemotherapy and cancer have resulted in you having no white blood cells. These are the cells that can fight pneumonia. Our antibiotics alone cannot fix this without help from your white blood cells." He glanced to his left to look at his wife.

"I hate to say it, but there's almost no chance that this pneumonia will go away, but I will admit you to the hospital, if you wish, to keep you comfortable and pain-free," I explained. They both nodded their understanding.

"One important issue to discuss is what your wishes are if your heart stops. We don't have to shock you and do chest compressions, which hurts a lot if you don't want us to. I want to know what your wishes are."

His wife looked confused, but he made his wishes crystal clear when he grabbed my hand. "I want you to do everything you can," he pleaded.

It shocked me. I did not expect or want this response.

"Absolutely, sir. We will do it if you wish. I want to make sure that you're both aware that it will hurt, and that I expect that we will find a need to do it in the next day or so. There does not appear to be much chance that you will recover from this most recent, horrible lung infection," I repeated as sincerely as I could.

"Do what you can, Doc. I am not ready to die yet."

I patted his hand and squeezed his wife's other hand.

"I'll write up his admission orders and arrange for a bed in our ICU. It will take time. Perhaps you can join your family in our waiting room? We will let you all know when he's ready to go upstairs," I suggested. She agreed and left to join a large family gathering. They all knew that the end was near. She needed to tell them of my new, final prognosis.

"Doctor Adams, we need you in bed three," announced the nurse. "His heart has stopped."

It had been ten minutes since his wife had left. I was writing the admission orders.

"OK. Do me a favor and see if there are any nurses or students that need experience with a full code. Then call the code to bed three, please."

"What? Are you telling me he's a full code?" she whispered incredulously.

"Yes, he is. He made his wishes clear, and his wife agreed. There's no chance that it will save him, so take your time, but gather the code team please. I will be right there."

We ran the code. I intubated him and had the nurse begin artificial respirations with the attached blue bag. We gave cardiac drugs that stimulated his heart and we shocked him five times. Multiple members of the team rotated giving chest compressions. The first three shocks brought back a dysfunctional heartbeat for a few seconds. We ran through the entire gamut of drugs available, per protocol, and shocked him again.

"Can anyone think of anything we have not done?" I solicited. There was no response.

"Please clean him up. Leave the endotracheal tube in his throat for now, until I find out if the family wants an autopsy. I'm going to the waiting room to speak with the family," I concluded, with sadness in my voice. There were a few tears, as always, in the team's eyes.

Death was always difficult, even when expected.

Chapter 40 – 82nd Airborne Clinic Lessons

One of my more rewarding jobs as a doctor was as the Clinic Commander of the 82nd Airborne Division's Robinson Health Clinic. The clinic was named after General Roscoe Robinson, Jr., the first African American four-star general in the U.S. Army. He was a West Point graduate, and he had commanded the Division in 1976.

We cared for 12,000 division officers, enlisted men, and their families. There were six family physicians and eighteen physician assistants or nurse practitioners assigned to the clinic. The administrative and nursing staff were mostly civilian employees.

I spent half my time seeing patients and the other half handling administrative and command issues. We managed our pregnant patients, delivered their babies, and helped with all family medical needs. Our physician assistants (PAs) were often brand-new PA school graduates. They came in early and managed the active-duty sick call clinic. The staff would see numerous walk-in men and women with minor issues like colds, rashes, or pulled muscles.

After the often-crowded early morning sick call, the PAs would see scheduled patients for routine care. There were physicians present all the time that they could go to with questions, but they were always quite busy.

This led to a problem. When a PA or NP had a question, it was often difficult to get a doctor to pause seeing his scheduled clinic patients and go give a second opinion.

In my first month, I was presented with four cases of medical misdiagnoses to evaluate and manage. In one example, the error could easily have resulted in a malpractice claim. This was unacceptable.

I did something relatively unprecedented and implemented a physician Preceptor program. Each day, one physician was taken off the clinic schedule and assigned as Preceptor for the entire staff. Anyone with a question or concern could now find a doctor to help. Mistakes evaporated, education of our new wet-behind-the-ears physician extenders increased, and everyone benefitted.

We started receiving awards for excellence at an unprecedented rate. It got command attention. When our higher-ups came to find out what we were doing, they became slightly distressed to learn that one doctor a day was not seeing scheduled patients. This would, of course, impact productivity, they observed.

In most organizations, it is easier to receive forgiveness than to get permission. This new initiative would be challenged eventually, so I was ready.

The new program did not impact productivity, and it markedly improved patient and staff satisfaction. Our Preceptor could see walk-in patients when all the other appointments were full, and they did. A walk-in would gladly wait to be seen if the Preceptor was helping elsewhere. When a sick or worried patient comes to any clinic or ER, they are scared. Some believe the worst and worry they might die. Even a simple rash could mean a deadly disease if you check the Internet.

The hospital commander left satisfied but watchful.

A three-star general's wife came to see me one day. Five other physicians had seen her for several complaints. She had undergone surgery. Various specialists had scanned and scoped her, but she was still having problems.

"Doctor, I'm distraught. No one can tell me what's wrong with me. I'm in pain all the time, and I can't sleep. I'm losing weight and have headaches often. My periods were awful, so they did a hysterectomy, and now I'm having hot flashes, and intercourse hurts. What's wrong with me?" she pleaded.

This was the wife of a general that I had been honored to serve before. Fort Bragg soldiers were at war. I needed to find the answer to her question. I had already read her chart with detailed notes from OB/GYN, gastroenterology, general surgery, dermatology, internal medicine, physical therapy, and neurology. Senior physicians had seen her in each department and had done what they thought best for the symptom they were evaluating. She was the general's wife, after all.

I knew, almost for sure, what her problem was, and I walked her down that path. After we had reviewed all her symptoms and her failed treatments, she was in tears.

"I need to apologize to you for it taking so long for you to get here," I whispered.

"I can help you with all your problems. Your issue is not bad or dangerous. You're not going to die. All your symptoms are commonly seen in men and women in stressful situations. As the spouse of a commander at war, your stress levels are unmeasurable. Stress affects every organ system in the body," I concluded after a long, detailed discussion.

I had her attention now.

"I would like to start you on a nightly pill for depression that will work fairly soon and help you with sleep, memory, energy, and even your sex life. I want to give your husband back the woman he married," I finished with a smile.

She nodded and dried her tears. She had already figured this out, but no one had yet given her permission to address it. I wrote a prescription, filled it at our on-site pharmacy, and escorted her to her car.

"I would like your permission to share our conversation with your husband. My explaining to you that you have had a lot of unnecessary attention, and maybe even surgery you did not need, will be hard for me to explain. I hope you will let me do that?" I questioned.

"Of course," she replied, and there was hope in her voice.

I was able to see the general immediately by mentioning his wife and my role. We sat in his huge conference room at a long polished wooden table that sat at least twenty-five people. Just the two of us. It was intimidating.

After a summary of my visit with his wife, and a repeat of my belief that I would make her better soon, I concluded, "So, sir, when she left today, I promised her I would give you back the woman you married."

The general had not uttered a word in the ten minutes it took me to get to the conclusion. He had listened judiciously.

He leaned back in his chair, fixed me with his eyes, and asked, "One question Doc. What makes you right, and all those other doctors wrong?"

Wow. He nailed it. That is why he's the general.

I spent the next few minutes answering that question by explaining that our medical system is carved into lots of little boxes. Doctors lived and worked well in their small boxes. They rarely stepped outside of their individual ability areas. Only one specialty worked in all those different boxes. Family Medicine physicians were trained in and worked in all the boxes.

I concluded by repeating that I was sure I was right. I would see her again in one month, and she would be better. "I told your wife I was certain she would feel better, and I told her I liked chocolate chip cookies," I concluded with a self-confidence I hoped he saw.

One month later, she came back to see me escorted by her smiling husband, who carried a tray of freshly baked chocolate chip cookies.

My Preceptor system worked. For the next two years, we became the best clinic on Fort Bragg. I had a reserved parking spot at the hospital for nine months in a row. The sign said, "Reserved, Clinic of the Month."

All the family physicians assigned to the clinic delivered the pregnant patients they followed. It was the best of all worlds for the family and for the doctor. We practiced *womb to tomb* care. We followed the pregnancy, delivered the child, cared for the entire family, and held the hands of our older patients when they died.

At eighteen years old, my son was considering going to medical school to follow in my footsteps. He had seen my joy and listened to my stories of new life. He asked to see a birth with me, so I told him I would look for an opportunity. One presented a few months later.

"Trey, if you still want to see a birth, tonight is a good time," I said, by phone. It was 11 PM on a Friday. He was a senior in high school.

"Yes, Dad. I guess so. What should I do?" he asked tentatively.

"I have asked the couple if they would let you watch. They said *yes*. We will be delivering in about an hour. Come up to the labor deck and ask for me. We have begun the pushing phase, so we will have a baby soon. Park in the front lot, and take the elevators to the third floor," I finished.

He arrived thirty minutes later, dressed in khaki slacks and a yellow polo shirt, looking nervous. I introduced him to the couple, as the soon-to-be mother began another contraction. She nodded at the quick introduction.

"Trey stand in the corner over there and watch. I'll be talking to them, so you can hear what's going on too."

He nodded and moved silently to the corner with the best view.

The nurse and the father stood to my right. I took the official and customary position at the foot of the bed between the mother's spread and bent legs. "You are doing great," I encouraged.

Dad was wide-eyed, and the nurse was watching the monitor. Mom had an epidural and could not sense the contractions, so the monitor told us when she needed to push. The head was making an appearance.

"OK, here he comes," I whispered. "Keep the pushing going, please."

I placed my fingers on the emerging head to control the rate of progress. I watched the vaginal skin surrounding the head as it stretched to allow passage. It did not look like I would need to cut an episiotomy to make room, but I could see a small tear beginning in the vaginal skin. I could sew that up later if needed.

The head slowly emerged. A gush of clear fluid and whitish tissue followed it. The body rotated, as desired, and the rest of the baby flowed wetly into my waiting hands. The bluish umbilical cord stretched from the baby to the now-closed vaginal opening.

"Oh, wow!" whispered our amazed observer in the corner.

"It's a girl," I announced smiling.

Chapter 41 - Stress Kills

Fort Bragg had lots of general officers, and they were waging war. A 3-star general is a Lieutenant General. He had a full-time aide who called me one afternoon to ask if the general could see me at 5 PM.

His aide and I already knew that the only answer to the question he was asking was, "Yes, sir!"

It was approaching our five o'clock closing time, but the general was coming.

I grabbed my senior enlisted NCOIC (Non-commissioned Officer In Charge) and Clinic Administrator and requested them to stay until the general came. I might need them. They willingly agreed.

The general's Humvee pulled up in front. It was camouflage brown and had a 3-star license plate. The driver Aide got out to get the passenger door open, but out popped his charge. He walked purposefully through the double glass doors and found me waiting in the entry area.

My NCOIC and Administrator were watching from the adjoining office hallway.

He stuck his hand out and smiled. "Doc, I think I'm depressed," he stated, so only I could hear.

"One moment, sir, and we will head back to an exam room," I responded.

"You all can head home," I said to my waiting staff. "I've got this."

They nodded, and I turned to my patient. I had been his doctor in the past when he was in another job.

"Sir, you have already made the diagnosis for me. Why don't we move to my office and discuss how I can help?"

He left after thirty minutes with medication, reassurance and a follow-up plan.

If a male patient thinks he is depressed, he probably is. Men do not like to admit it. Women are easier to diagnose because they cry.

When a man who society has taught not to cry or display soft emotions is depressed, he presents differently. Men will willingly report memory problems, anger issues, and sleep disturbances. Commonly, a man will present with an ache or pain that makes little sense. It is just an excuse to see the doctor.

After a careful exam finding nothing significant or observing an exaggerated response to my exam, I take a moment to acknowledge the presenting issue and redirect the conversation.

"Your elbow should get better with ice and ibuprofen," I start. "Have you had any falls or heavy lifting recently? Is there anything else bothering you, like sleep or memory?" I like to slip in.

"Wow, you got that. My memory is gone," is a frequent reply.

"Are you having any anger or sleep issues?" I usually ask.

When the answer is yes to either of these, the diagnosis is clear.

"If I can give you a pill that you take once a day, and it will make your memory, sleep, and anger issues better, would you take it?"

"Absolutely," is the usual grateful response.

"There's a hormone in the brain that is altered by stress. The pill I will give you resets the happy pathways. If you look it up, they label it as an antidepressant, but that is an old-fashioned term we used before we discovered these neurotransmitters in the brain."

This approach avoids the typical male tendency to refuse to admit what they perceive as a weakness called depression. I emphasize the positive benefits. The result, in a few weeks, is always gratifying.

As is always the case in the military, there came a time for me to move on. I went to Iraq, and those in charge directed subsequent clinic commanders to increase productivity with fewer available doctors. They had scrapped the Preceptor system. When I returned a year later, the staff informed me their operation was in trouble again. No more awards. Few leaders remained that had learned from what we had done. It made me sad.

Chapter 42 – DELTA Force Doc – Can You Save The Hand?

After two years of working at Fort Bragg, NC, as a Clinic Director, I was approached by the secret DELTA Force organization. They asked me to apply for the job of the unit's Command Surgeon. "Surgeon" is a military title given to physicians of any specialty when assigned to a medical command and staff position in the military. As a family physician, I was invited to become the senior medical advisor to the commander.

I was recruited in part because of my past special operations experience. I accepted the position and reported to the Deputy Commander's office for my initial brief.

"Doc," pronounced the intent colonel. "I've done the job of every officer on my staff, except yours. I can never do your job, but I consider it essential to our command's success. I want you to provide the best medical care in the military to my staff and their families. I'll expect you to ask for what you need to accomplish this, and when you ask me, I will approve it every time. I'm not qualified to argue with you, so if you say we need it, you'll get it."

That promise was never broken. Our clinic building was expanded and renamed in honor of unit medics killed in combat. Then we opened the doors to family members. We added a dental clinic, provided obstetrics care and began delivering the children of unit moms. I delivered forty-four babies for these families. When I return now for reunion gatherings, there is always a mom or dad that regales me with stories of their children that I delivered. Good times.

Challenging patients frequently presented because of the constant training with live weapons, explosive ordinance, parachuting, and aviation operations.

"Eagle down," came the message to my secure phone. "There has been an accident in the field with an explosive injury to a hand. He's en route to the hospital now," finished the voice on my secure phone.

"Roger that. I'm on my way. Give me his name, please."

The name was passed, and as many times before, I drove above the speed limit to the emergency room. I arrived soon after the casualty did and was met by the nurse, who expected me.

"Hello, Doctor Adams," she breathed. "Your patient is in room three. He may have lost his hand."

"Thank you," I replied. "How is he doing?"

"Sir, I have to be honest with you. He ought to be screaming in pain. His hand is almost completely gone! But he is just looking at it, while we clean it, and asking if we can save it. Who is this man?" She finished in awe.

He's the definition of someone special. "He's made of different stuff," I replied.

When I got to the room, he was looking at his hand. Most of the soft tissue was gone. Bones of his fingers were mostly there, but he could not move them. There were burned edges of flesh visible down to the wrist area.

I had been briefed en route, by the medic on the scene, that the squad was conducting simulated combat building clearance operations. He had pulled the pin on a flash-bang grenade to throw forward. Instead of the standard three-second delay, it had detonated instantly in his hand. A flash-bang grenade produces a brilliant, eye-blinding flash of light and heat, with a loud explosive noise, but does not produce shrapnel. It is used to disorient attackers before entering a room.

The orthopedic hand surgeon arrived almost immediately after we called him. He took a careful look and directed us to move to the operating room. He would be better able to determine the extent of the injury with the patient under anesthesia. Our patient insisted on a local nerve block so he could listen and watch.

Who were these men, and where do we get them?

A few months later, after they had fitted him with a new functional artificial hand, he came to me and requested to be medically cleared to freefall parachute again.

Where do these men come from?

The next week the same orthopedic medical team was back in the operating room. During building assault training, a rope rappelling rig had failed, and my new patient had slid down a four-story building. He had landed feet first onto the ground and performed the best parachute-landing fall he could. His feet took the brunt of the fall, absorbing the impact of full body weight, weapon, and backpack. He had broken almost every bone in his two feet. We were passing stainless steel wires from the tip of each toe back towards the heel as we manually pushed bone fragments back in line.

"Bob, I hate to hang black crepe here," stated the concerned surgeon. "These wires pass through the smooth cartilage of every joint in his toes and feet, and this creates a type of joint arthritis that will probably make it impossible to run again. Walking will be painful for a long time."

"Thanks, Kurt," I replied, concerned. "I'll let the boss know."

That afternoon, after seeing our patient tucked in and stable, I went back to the unit and passed the same prognostic information to the commander.

"Really, Doc?" he responded. "I know you're telling me what *the book* says, but I'll suggest something different. He'll be running in six months," he predicted, smiling.

"You just don't know yet what these men are made of," he concluded.

Six months later, I watched him run by the clinic and wave.

Chapter 43 – Freefall Hero – Resuscitation and NSAIDs

A freefall parachutist glided precisely to the target area where a bright orange "T" was placed. A medic watched. Today was a routine daylight freefall parachute jump event, and all was going without a hitch.

The parachutist stalled his chute as he approached the landing area. It would allow for a soft, controlled stand-up landing. His feet touched, and he collapsed and rolled on his side.

The surprised medic trotted over. "Are you OK?" he asked.

"I'm OK, Doc. Thanks. I hurt my hip when the chute opened, and it's still pretty tender," he grumbled.

"You might want to let us look at that. Let me get you to the clinic for a better look," stated the concerned medic.

"No. Really, I feel OK. Let me get the chute packed and back to the riggers shop. I'll do chute shake-out and then walk over to the clinic. I promise," he finished.

The medic had already informed me the patient was coming before he hobbled in. I planned to do a pelvic X-ray to be thorough.

"Lie back on the table for me," I requested.

The exam revealed a tender pelvic bone in the middle and the left side. When I put pressure on the hip bones, I could feel a slight movement and a crunching sensation. That could indicate a pelvic fracture. The pelvic bones come together to form an oval circle. If it breaks, it almost always breaks in two separate places.

"Let's get an X-ray. You might have broken your pelvic bone," I directed.

"Sure, Doc. But I think I pulled a muscle when the chute snapped open," he said somewhat confidently.

He stood up and walked to the wall where the X-ray display was. He had been here before.

With him standing against the X-ray table, hands over his head, we took two pictures.

"I don't see an obvious fracture," I stated, confused.

"I still think you may have fractured your pelvis. I want you to go to the ER, and I will have our orthopedic doctor look at you," I concluded.

"Seriously, Doc? It's five o'clock, and I need to get home. It doesn't hurt that bad. I promise I will go get it looked at in the morning if you let me go home today," he pleaded.

"Fine. But you can't drive, so I'll have our medic take you home and pick you up in the morning. He'll take you to the ortho clinic. OK?" I said, knowing, in my heart, I was making a mistake.

I finished some chart notes and reached for my jacket.

My phone rang. It was the medic.

"Doc," he panted. "I think he's dead. I'm doing CPR on the sidewalk to his house. He collapsed."

"Damn! I knew it!" I started. "He has a broken pelvis, and he's bleeding internally. I have the address, and I will call 911. Take him to the civilian hospital near you," I panted. "I'll call you right back."

The ambulance crew was five minutes away. I redialed the medic.

"Doc, he's awake now. He collapsed and seemed to stop breathing. I have my bag in the car if you want me to start an IV?" he asked.

"He needs fluids, but is that the ambulance siren I hear?"

"It is, sir. I'll let them know you think he has a broken pelvis and is bleeding internally. Gotta go, sir. I'll call you from the hospital," he concluded.

Son of a bitch! I knew it. I let him talk me out of doing the safe thing. Damn.

The report from the medic that night noted he had indeed broken his pelvis in two places. It was apparent on the X-ray taken with him lying flat. When we took the X-ray with him standing, the bones were pushed back into place by gravity, and the fracture was not as visible.

He was lucky. The pelvis filled up with blood and formed a clot the size of a small basketball. This put internal pressure on the leaking vessels and stopped the blood flow. Surgery was not needed, and he was discharged two days later. Light duty was ordered, and ibuprofen was given for pain. The medic took him home, and he was back at work in a week.

Six weeks later, he was out in the field again, walking without pain.

Training events always had a medic assigned. This day was no different, and the same medic oversaw the activity.

"Jim," the medic began, "Are you feeling OK? You look pale. Is anything wrong?"

"Not really. I've been a bit weak for some reason. I have been taking the ibuprofen three times a day like the ortho doc told me," he observed.

"Whoa. Have you been taking that medicine for six weeks now?" began the now more attentive medic.

"Are you having any other symptoms, like acid indigestion?" he continued.

"A bit, yes, but I have noticed my stools have turned into a black tarry mess the last three days," he stated conversationally.

The medic brought him to me, noting that he might have a bleeding ulcer. He did, and we admitted him to the hospital again. He needed a transfusion to get his blood count back to an acceptable level. The ibuprofen should have been stopped long ago, as it frequently causes bleeding if taken daily for long periods.

A month later, the trooper returned for a recheck.

"Doc, I would like you to remove the restriction for me about freefall parachuting, please," he started.

I had expected this. "Jim, you're forty-five years old. You almost died twice. You have tempted fate one too many times. I am sorry, but you need to give up parachute operations," I stated as powerfully and compassionately as I could.

"Well, I had to ask," he stated, smiling. He had been pretty sure I would say no.

Chapter 44 – Don't Do Anything Strenuous!

"Doc, Eagle down," came the radio call. It was 2 AM, and we were in the middle of a combat training exercise.

"It's the Commander," came the next squawk. "He's been shot in the eye."

We were using rubber bullets and non-fragmenting flash-bang grenades, but these devices were frequent causes of training injuries. The eye was a very vulnerable organ.

"Transport to the clinic, I'm on the way now," I replied with a shaky voice. Visions of what I might see were flashing through my brain.

The ambulance and two medics arrived minutes after I did. We had an expertly capable clinic, with an urgent care slit lamp for examining eyes.

The "boss" was a full bird colonel, and he commanded the best of the best in Special Forces operators. He had not been wearing his safety glasses, and a ricochet rubber bullet had hit him square in the left eye. A bruise on the eyelid suggested he had closed his eye in time.

I completed the eye exam after adding eye drops to numb the pain. This allowed him to open his eye while I glanced through the slit lamp. The lamp lighted and magnified the entire eyeball.

"Sir, can you see out of your left eye?"

"I see light, Doc. Not much else. It gets brighter when you move that gadget of yours," he grumbled. He was an intimidating combat veteran, and he wanted it that way.

"Sir, it appears you have a burst of the globe of your eyeball. There's a small amount of the vitreous jelly leaking out. I'll put a patch over your eye and wrap your head to hold it in place and call our eye surgeon to meet us in the emergency room. You might need surgery," I stated less than confidently.

The on-call ophthalmologist met us in the emergency room. He had come in from home and looked tired. Once I unwrapped the dressing, he was all business.

'Wow, that is interesting," he started. "The globe is definitely ruptured, and the vitreous is filled with blood. This is not a penetrating wound, so a foreign body is unlikely," he instructed.

"The white area of your eye, sir, has an impressive burst defect in it. Some vitreous and blood leaked, but not much. Often, we need to sew the defect closed, but in your case, the sclera has burst open in this small area such that there are multiple edges, like a starburst. It looks like the sudden impact of the rubber bullet caused the eyeball to pop like a pimple might do," he continued.

"I'll numb it again and push the ruptured tissue back in place. Doing this will avoid the need for surgery. It will be important for you to avoid any physical activity that could raise the pressure in your eye. Exercise of any kind is bad," he finished.

His patient nodded and growled, "I can do desk work, right, Doc?"

"Yes, sir. I would like to see you back in my office in two days, please. But, if you have any worsening pain or flashing lights in that eye, please let Doctor Adams know, and I will see you right away. Flashing lights can be a sign of a detaching retina in the back of your eye, and that causes blindness if not caught and fixed early."

"As a reminder," he continued, "there's lots of blood in the vitreous jelly of your eye. That should reabsorb over the next few days. As it does, your vision will return. The eye is self-cleaning, and it will get rid of the blood. You'll notice floaters in your visual field at times. These are blood cells suspended and moving around in the jelly."

A week later, on Sunday night after dinner, the commander called me.

"Doc, I can't see out of my left eye again," was all he said.

"Did you do anything strenuous this weekend, sir?" I asked warily.

"No, nothing."

"Roger that, sir. Head for the emergency room again, please. The ophthalmologist and I will meet you there. Please have someone drive you," I finished.

In the ER eye exam area, the ophthalmologist completed his exam once again.

"I'm not sure why, but the vitreous is filled with blood again. I could go in and try to vacuum it out, but it cleared OK last week. I want to avoid sticking a needle in there, so let's watch it again and expect it to clear. I can't overemphasize the need to take it easy, sir."

The boss grunted. His teenage daughter escorted him back to their car.

Monday morning found him at work as usual. After completing my morning office visits, I walked across the parking area to the command suite. His secretary escorted me in. He had removed his patch and was scribbling on paperwork.

"How's the eye this morning, sir? Any pain?" I started.

"Still blind as a bat, Doc. No pain," he grumbled, looking at me unhappily.

I did a quick exam with my light and decided everything was as expected. I reminded him to take it easy and let myself out.

His secretary was waiting for me.

"Hey Doc, did the colonel, by any chance, tell you he went freefall parachuting on Friday?" she added with wide questioning eyes.

The commander's secretary was legendary in the command and had served many past commanders. Everyone loved her, and she remained as committed to the mission as any shooter on the compound.

"He did what?!" I exclaimed, choking back disbelief. She nodded.

I spun around and slid back into the CO's office. He had overheard our exchange.

"You did what?" I started in an unbelieving tone.

"Now, Doc, take it easy. Freefall is not that strenuous," he stated guiltily.

"Of course, you're correct, sir -- until you pull the ripcord at 120 miles an hour and get whipped upright in the harness," I growled with a glare.

I now understood why he had called me on Sunday. He had gone blind again after the jump and had been hoping it would clear up. When it did not, after two days, he decided to call.

Damn.

I missed that one.

Chapter 45 - Charity Hospital Gunshots

"There had been 1,669 gunshot-wound patients seen in the Charity Hospital emergency room in the two years before I wrote that article. We had a seventy-seven percent survival rate," stated my host with pride. I was holding an article he had authored and published. This was the start of my gunshot-wound training week in New Orleans. We had researched the best place for learning and had set up a formal training agreement between the Army and Charity Hospital. Our doctors and medics would rotate there to get real-world experience.

There was a reason why so many were seen at this one hospital. At this time, in 1999, Louisiana had universal health insurance for anyone in the state - resident or visitor. As a result, they controlled the system. If you got shot in New Orleans, you were going to Charity Hospital. They were the best, and you were given no other options.

Doctor Kennan Buechter was the Chief of Trauma Surgery at Charity Hospital, where it was possible to see ten to fifteen gunshot wounds a day.

I was a guest at his pool for a dinner of 'Turducken.' This New Orleans specialty was roasting over an open fire. It consisted of a turkey, stuffed with a duck, stuffed with a chicken. Tur-duck-en. It smelled delicious and tasted as good as I had hoped it would.

"My first shift in your ER is tonight, so I'll limit my Turducken feast to one beer," I said.

"Spoilsport," he smiled.

My beeper went off at 10:05 PM. So did fifteen other pagers. I was on the top floor of the ancient building, where visitors could bunk overnight on cots with thin mattresses. The trauma team was alerted that a gunshot was en route. What followed was well-rehearsed and reminded me of a ballet in surgical scrubs.

"We have two patients seven minutes out. Multiple wounds in both" stated the head nurse on the raised platform above the two-bed treatment area. She held the action-item checklist. IV bags and large bore needles were made ready, sterile urinary catheters were unwrapped, intubation trays were checked and made ready, and bed linens were pulled back to receive the casualties. Staff quickly moved to their pre-arranged positions. Everyone had a specific task.

Each patient would receive the same initial assessment. Blood would be drawn, IV access established in two extremities, a urinary catheter placed, and urine sampled for blood. Bleeding was stopped with pressure bandages, clothing was entirely removed with scissors, and findings were announced and recorded.

"GSW (*gunshot wound*) entry wound times two right buttock, and GSW times one left buttock. No exit wound seen," announced the bed one doctor who had received the first casualty. Casualty number two arrived.

"Don't pay any attention to the two bullets in my abdomen," stated the second patient. "Those are old. Leftover from last time."

"OK, bed two is talking, and his leg wound bleeding is controlled. Cath-urine and blood samples are obtained. Take him to X-ray first, please," stated the doctor coolly.

"What about some morphine?" asked our charge as he rolled out the door.

"Not yet, sir. We need to see your lung X-ray first."

The patient groaned unhappily as he was rolled out the door.

Within minutes after arrival, both men had been assessed, sampled, stripped, cleaned, and treated for the initial findings.

"How did you get shot in the butt? The angle of entry is unusual," noted the doctor at bed one.

"They were shooting at us from the street in front of us. I was climbing over the front seat to the back when I got hit," he moaned.

Later that evening, I was helping the fifth casualty of the night. His single-gunshot right side wound had caused one lung to collapse due to a pneumothorax. The X-ray showed the bullet in his abdomen. It likely nicked the lung, which sat on the diaphragm. A pneumothorax is created when each breath allows more air to leak into the space between the chest wall and the lining of the lung. It hurt, and it was pushing the lung into a smaller space with each breath. It was my first chance to insert a chest tube.

"I know where it goes and how to suture it in place," I explained to the trauma resident.

"Go ahead and do it then," he directed. We were in the X-ray room, looking at the collapsing lung picture. I walked back to the patient and found the nurse. She already had the chest tube set open and bedside.

"Raise the bed to thirty degrees, please," I requested of the nurse.

"Sir, I'm going to numb the skin on your side under your arm here. Please place your arm on your head and keep it there. In a few seconds, it will be numb, and I'll insert a tube into the lung area to let the air out that is collapsing your lung. You will breathe better after the air comes out," I finished assertively.

"Do it, Doc. I can't breathe."

I felt for the space between his ribs, midway up the chest, and injected five cc's of the numbing medicine. It worked in seconds, so I grabbed the knife and cut a deep ½ inch incision through the skin. The patient had his arm on his head and watched intently.

The nurse handed me the large-bore chest tube. I lined it up to go deep and up toward his armpit and pushed hard but did not get penetration. I pushed harder and sensed the tube advance.

"Ow, shit, Doc. That hurts!"

I did not hear the rush of air I expected, but we could see that the tube was in place. I sutured it as planned and asked the nurse to take him to X-ray to confirm placement and reduction of the air space.

"Did you hear a rush of air?" asked the trauma surgeon as we analyzed the X-ray.

"No, but it went in all the way," I mumbled.

"Well, you did not puncture the pleural lining, so it's under his ribs but not in the lung space. Go pull it out and do it again. This time go straight in until you hear the air. Then you can angle it up and suture it back in place. Got it?"

"Yes, sir, and thank you. I need to do this," I stated.

With the knowledge of what I had done wrong, and with the gentle encouragement of the nurse, the tube popped neatly through the tough pleural lung lining. We both smiled at the large rush of air whooshing out the tube.

The patient's face showed relief as he took a deeper breath.

The next stop was the operating room. I followed the gurney up two floors. It was 2 AM, and the surgeon on call was Doctor Buechter himself. I was in the presence of greatness, so I scrubbed in gratefully and joined Doctor Buechter and one of his residents at the OR table.

"Would you like to open him up?" probed Doctor Buechter. The patient was asleep under anesthesia, and we were planning to do an exploration of the entire abdomen. The bullet was in there somewhere. Removing it was not the issue. We needed to find out what internal organs it had perforated and fix those. Bowel perforation can lead to infection and death. The liver, spleen, and kidneys do not respond well to bullets passing through them.

I nodded, yes. "If you will show me where to cut."

"Knife to Doctor Adams," he directed as he plopped the blade into my outstretched hand.

He used his gloved hand to draw a line from below the diaphragm, down and around the belly button, to four inches below that. I could see it as a dotted line in my mind.

The incision began where directed, and I pushed with enough force to separate the skin down to the layer of yellow subcutaneous fat. That was a feat of some significance for a non-surgery-trained physician. I was pleased.

As the knife approached the belly button, I paused to make a turn with the knife. Bad decision. Lifting the blade and turning it to continue caused a tiny break in the smooth line of separated flesh. I left a 'rabbit ear' defect in the otherwise gorgeous incision. This earned me a glance from the watching resident and my mentor, but no grunt or sound followed. They had both done it in their inexperienced surgical days. We would all remember and proceed differently in the future.

We found the bullet by feel. It was embedded in deep tissue below the layers of intact bowel and had not perforated a single organ or vessel. Both surgeons tried to prove that finding wrong as they ran fingers along bowel and organs. They agreed that all we needed to do was to close him up. The bullet stayed where it was. Dissecting deeper to get it could cause more damage.

Closing the long, slightly imperfect incision took a few minutes. A staple gun was produced, and I was allowed to pull the skin edges together with forceps while the resident neatly and accurately placed shiny steel staples every centimeter from bottom to top.

He graciously placed my small rabbit ear defect in the middle of one staple.

"War is an ugly thing, but not the ugliest of things. The decayed and degraded state of moral and patriotic feeling, which thinks that nothing is worth war is much worse.
The person who has nothing for which he is willing to fight, nothing which is more important than his own personal safety, is a miserable creature and has no chance of being free unless made and kept so by the exertions of better men than himself." John Stuart Mill

WARTIME PHYSICIAN

Chapter 46 – Habbaniya, Iraq – Water Bottle Showers

After almost four years with DELTA, I returned to a more traditional job as a family physician and again as the 82nd Airborne Clinic Commander, and now wore the rank of Colonel.

Then we invaded Iraq for the second time.

I volunteered to go early in the conflict to lock in a six-month deployment. All doctors would need to go eventually, and it appeared future deployments would be one year long.

At my request, they assigned me to the 82nd Airborne Division, 782nd Battalion, Charlie Medical Company. They were deploying soon to Habbaniya, Iraq, for combat operations.

The advance party arrived in the war zone by air via the safer, sweltering country of Kuwait. It was 130 degrees outside, and the air was so dry it burned one's mouth and nose to breathe it. A local store was taking our standard-issue t-shirts, cutting them, and making round neck gaiters we could pull over our heads and wear as face masks. These repurposed t-shirts filtered the dust and held enough moisture from our breath to cool the air we sucked slowly into our lungs.

Our final destination in Iraq was an abandoned bombed-out airfield. It had been the site of a battle in WW II when it functioned as a British RAF military airfield. Now it was covered with bomb craters, ruined aircraft, and empty buildings or hangars. The locals had scavenged all the glass, doors, and internal wiring. Stone buildings stood empty with six inches of brown sand and dust on the floors.

There were only two colors visible anywhere. The buildings and sand were brown. Everywhere was brown, our uniforms were brown. Even our teeth were brown from the omnipresent dust swirling around us. The other color was the blue of the sky.

After months in a colorless environment, the rods and cones of our retinas changed. They turned themselves partially off. When we returned, many months later, to a world with color, we would all notice that greens and reds appeared markedly different. Trees and brick houses glowed with vibrant, more profound, richer colors. The retina had to readjust again to process the explosions of color, not viewed in a long time.

We came into possession of naked building remnants and were told to make them livable. The main fighting force would be arriving in a few days. There was trash everywhere, and we had no power or water. We had our hands, brooms, and shovels, and one generator to provide light in the evenings. We ate MREs (meals ready to eat) in heavy plastic bags and drank water from cases of quart-sized plastic bottles. The empty bottles blew away, and we began to call them the 'national flower of Iraq,' as they tumbled along the desert sands.

A shower at the end of a day was comprised of two quart-sized bottles of water poured over a naked body. At first, we thought a towel would be needed. But, as fast as the water rolled down our bodies, and we rubbed quickly with our hands, it evaporated. We were dry seconds after rubbing the wet brownish water off our dust-covered nudity.

I was given charge of a five-room building that had an old medical red cross painted on an inside wall. It was to become the Division Support Command clinic and emergency room. We began by sweeping out the dense layer of dirt and dust that had settled onto the floor and every corner of each room. The toilet area comprised two holes in the floor. We plugged the holes and filled them with sand, and the incessant flies went away.

There was a small, single-room building close by that had been used for Iraqi chemical warfare training. It was covered with old gas masks, needles with a chemical antidote, and reeked faintly of tear gas. We placed it off-limits. Later we would bring in fire trucks to wash the entire building and surrounding area.

The local population jumped at the chance to earn cash, so we hired men to make and install plywood doors and windows. We needed to keep the sand out. A generator provided lighting. The "Med Shed" had the highest priority for light, and eventually, weeks later, air conditioning.

We all lost weight. Our desert-colored camouflage uniforms had streaks of white salt all over them. We drank water regularly, and sweat poured out of us, unseen and unnoticed. The air was so arid that sweat evaporated before it could even form a film on our skin. The clothing acted as a filter, and the salt was captured in the cloth as sweat evaporated. That created the white salt streaks. We could see and taste the salt caked onto our clothing.

Weeks later, we got a portable air conditioning unit. We needed it to care for our sick patients. There was a five-bed holding area, a two-room operating and casualty treatment area, a portable X-ray machine, and a tiny lab/pharmacy. The heat had severely degraded the medical supplies, injectables medications, and test kits. They had been transported and stored in metal Conex boxes sitting in the sun, where internal temperatures exceeded 200 degrees.

The Division and other units ran daily combat missions in our area, and we supplied ambulance and medic coverage to their convoys. Specialist Nathaniel Haney was the same age as my son. At eighteen years old, he was ready for war and had joined from Florida, right after high school. As a lean and lanky teen, he had no problem with the physical demands of jump school and the 82nd Airborne.

"Doc, I want to go on the convoy today," he pleaded.

"Haney, you're on the list. Don't worry. Your time is coming," I replied. In fact, I did not want to send him in harm's way. I delayed because he reminded me of my son. Then the war came right to us.

2 November 2003.

"Sir, there has been a CH-47 helo crash close by. They're asking for all available medical personnel," stated the out-of-breath runner from headquarters. The CH-47 was our biggest helicopter, and it could hold up to fifty-five passengers. These tired combatants were going to Kuwait for a mid-tour trip back home. Their bags were packed with gifts for family members.

"Where is this?" I queried. The runner pointed to the sky, where a dark line of smoke was visible.

"Sir, we have more vehicles coming. You will need to send your ambulances, medics, and doctors. There are bad roads in that area, but we will lead the way there," he shouted wide-eyed.

The medics were already scrambling for their aid bags. The three other doctors came towards me carrying helmets and putting on flak jackets.

"OK, Doctors Dobson and Healy can go forward with the medics. Each of you take an ambulance and some medics. Mary and I will stay here to set up the Emergency Room to receive casualties."

Doctor Mary Conlan was a Major and an experienced family physician. She moved to the trauma room, grabbed a medic, and started to set it up for receiving serious casualties.

"All I know so far is that it was a CH-47 with our unit folks on it. They were hit by an RPG rocket and went down. There's another CH-47 on site that was following. Their passengers are on the ground to help." *Oh no!*

I watched through the open clinic window as Medical Specialist Haney jumped into the last ambulance.

The scene was horrendous. There were twelve dead and twenty-four wounded. The bird was on fire, and men were trapped under its crumpled metal fuselage. Area support staff and medics tried to keep the fire away, while others crawled under bent metal to render aid. Bodies needed to be moved, bleeding stopped, burns bandaged, wounds cleaned with bottled water, and the disoriented moved to safety. The process lasted a long and individually challenging time.

Later, I saw Haney walking toward me. Hours had passed since he left. He was walking slowly and staring straight ahead. He walked past me without looking.

"Haney, how are you? How was it?" I asked softly as he passed.

He stopped, glanced back, and seemed to take a moment to focus on me and what I had asked. His face was pale and streaked by sweat and fine desert dust.

"Oh, hi Doc, I'm sorry." There was a quiet pause as he thought about how to answer me.

"That was not what I was expecting," he almost whispered.

The sadness and shock in his voice became life-altering. He would go on to do great things as a medic and a soldier, but he would never again be the same.

Chapter 47 - Flight Surgeons Flying

Flight Surgeons wear a well-earned silver badge on their uniforms. It designates us as qualified to treat our large and diverse aviation force. Flight surgeons go to school to learn aviation medicine, aeromedical policies and procedures, and to get stick time flying helicopters or flight simulators.

There is a financial incentive added to base pay for doctors that fly at least four hours a month. Flights can be in any military aircraft. MedEvac birds often operate with the flight doctors getting their flight time.

A war zone is different. MedEvac flights get shot at when they fly. I had wanted to sit on my helmet during my last MedEvac night flight. Red tracers from the enemy's AK-47 Kalashnikovs would streak by the open windows and doors. Imagining a lucky shot finding me from below was not a pretty thought.

As the senior doctor and flight surgeon, I would receive requests from nearby doctors to get flight time in our MedEvac birds. The previous month, a MedEvac helicopter had been shot down by a hand-fired RPG (rocket-propelled grenade). The two pilots died. One was a woman.

One of the doctors assigned to Habbaniya with me was a flight surgeon. She was the mother of two young children. She could use the extra $150 per month flight surgeon incentive pay.

I knew she would ask me again to fly. It was an unnecessary risk as I saw it. It bothered me when I flew, and it sucked that those with command authority did not see the inappropriateness of the regulation in a war zone.

"Dear LTG James Peake," read my email letter to the Surgeon General of the U.S. Army. I briefly outlined the issue. We had doctors in a war zone requesting to fly combat operations to get flight time. They needed four hours a month to earn the extra $150. The risk was not worth the pay, but our doctors were taking it to maintain their flight surgeon pay.

I pointed out that a soldier's combat pays only required that he or she be present in a combat zone. We did not need to shoot or get shot at to earn combat pay. The area soldiers and medical staff were all earning combat pay by just being in a combat zone.

Additionally, our combat pay and salary income were nontaxable for the months served in a combat zone. Families at home needed every extra penny to compensate for missing spouses and parents.

I concluded my missive with a request that he consider waiving the flight time requirement for doctors in a combat zone. My intuition hinted that no one had ever identified this issue. Our last shooting war was a long time ago.

The response from Washington was surprisingly quick. Lieutenant General Peake agreed and issued the order.

"Flight surgeons, in a war zone, are exempt from the flight hours required to earn flight pay." Signed, Lieutenant General James Peake, Army Surgeon General.

No doctors sustained injuries during flight operations while I was in Iraq. Thank you from all of us, General.

Chapter 48 – Iraq – Kidney Stones

"Doc! Just kill me, please!" cried the distressed helicopter pilot writhing on the exam table.

"Hang in there, Captain. I'm going to give you a shot that will help." He looked pitiful, but he was the second patient today with a kidney stone. We had seen almost one renal stone a day for the last few weeks. This was statistically very unusual. Something had to be causing it.

I gathered the other three doctors, and we tried to figure out what was going on. It did not take long.

"The one thing our patients have in common is they're in Iraq, in 130-degree heat, and are drinking water in large quantities," one doctor observed.

"Dehydration could be a factor, as water is leaving the body in unseen sweat as fast as it goes in," she continued.

"Wait a minute. Don't they add calcium and minerals to bottled water?" I began while grabbing an empty plastic bottle nearby. There was the answer. "Calcium chloride, sodium bicarbonate, and magnesium sulfate" were added to the water we were drinking in large quantities.

"This, plus the concentration that is occurring in the course of sweat evaporation, is causing kidney stones," I suggested. There were nods of agreement all around.

Our pediatrician said, "We need a different source of water. Why don't we start drinking from the water buffaloes outside? We use that water for washing. Let's start drinking it. I saw that they get it from the local Habbaniyah Lake and run it through a purifier. There are water buffaloes at each unit," he concluded. Water buffaloes were wheeled trailers holding 200 to 5000 gallons of water. They were pulled behind trucks and dropped off near our housing and clinic areas. They had gravity-fed nozzles and contained fresh water for cleaning and drinking.

I went to the senior officer in the headquarters nearby and presented our findings. He was aware his pilots were getting grounded for kidney stones, and other commands were reporting the same problem.

"Thank you, Doc. I will get the word out immediately, and we can increase local water production to meet the need. I hope you all are correct," he concluded.

"We will know in a few days, sir." We did know soon. The kidney stone problem evaporated like our sweat.

As I walked back, I tried to brush off the white stripes of salt that stained the front of my camouflage uniform. No luck.

A loud explosion nearby sucked out my air. It was nearby. Smoke and flames were erupting in a row of large tents set up in the area behind us. They were unoccupied.

I ran to the clinic and found the entire staff standing in the main hallway, and all dressed in their body armor, with helmets on. This was routine. We had mortar attacks in our area at random times. It was disconcerting.

Later that night, with just the duty staff now in the clinic, I picked up the one military phone we had and dialed stateside to a military hospital switchboard.

"Can you please connect me to this number?" I asked the operator and gave her my home phone number. I could not remember what time it would be in North Carolina, but it did not matter.

A call home was always welcome, and we always said the same things.

"Everything is fine here," I would begin. "Not much going on. Nothing for you to worry about."

Jeri would answer the same way. "We're all fine here. The kids are wonderful. No problems. Hurry home, and we love you." Always the same lies.

"Blam!" An explosion rocked our building.

"I gotta go, sweetheart. They're mortaring the clinic," I quickly said. As I hung up and reached for my helmet, I realized I had made a mistake. These were not the words I needed her to hear – ever.

I called back later that evening and tried to smooth over my mistake.

"No problem. I understand. Thanks for calling back. Nothing for you to worry about here either," she lied again. She was at her desk looking at the left upper corner of her computer screen where a constant video feed from Baghdad let her know if an explosion occurred.

We both went out of our way to paint a pretty picture, so neither of us would have more to stress over. It worked.

Chapter 49 - Mass Casualty

An ambulance roared up to the door a bit faster than usual. Out jumped two medics, and they moved to the rear doors.

"Doc! Mass casualty coming in. IED and vehicle rollover. We have two casualties on board, and one is bleeding badly. One more ambulance is coming," stated the medic on the passenger side of the dust-covered vehicle.

The medic hurried to the rear doors and swung them open. Another medic held pressure on a bloody wrapped leg wound. His eyes were wide and attentive.

Our medics appeared to grab the stretchers and move the first casualty inside. The injured trooper moaned, but I noticed a black "M" on his forehead. The medic had given him morphine for the pain. We had instructed all our combat medics in the proper use of injectable morphine, and they were authorized to carry it in the field.

The clinic staff was gathering to move casualties to one of our three rooms, as we had rehearsed. The first room was for 'Immediate' casualties needing airway or bleeding management. We set the next room up for 'Delayed' casualties who could wait until we handled the critical patients.

There were already two doctors in the first room, as the first casualty slid in the door on his stretcher. The stretcher dripped a trail of blood onto the floor.

"I'll take the Delayed room," I stated as I peeked in. "Do you need me here?"

"No, we've got this. Only two 'Immediates' now. Your room has four stretchers, and more medics are on the way," stated Mary, the triage physician.

The second ambulance arrived minutes later with four casualties onboard. We offloaded them to the Delayed room.

Military triage categorizes casualties into four types. DIME is the acronym. Delayed, Immediate, Minimal, and Expectant. Expectant is reserved for those with injuries so severe we do not expect them to survive.

I went to the first stretcher. It was set up off the floor between folding metal support legs. There were two medics there taking a history of the event. An IED had gone off after the vehicle they were in had passed. It caused rocks and shrapnel to hit their bodies and faces. Their flak vests had protected their trunk areas and were now lying on the floor by the stretchers.

The first man I came to lay flat on his back, peacefully relating the event and feeling lucky.

"All right, gents, let's do his exam by the book. Start at the head and work your way to his toes. Open his clothes and look for wounds," I directed. They looked intently, listened for heart and lung sounds, and palpated all the way down.

"Check for sensation and movement," I reminded them.

"Sir, would you wiggle your toes, please?" asked the medic. Nothing happened, and the patient looked confused.

I stepped to his feet and lightly stroked his toes on both feet.

"Sir, can you feel me touching your toes?" He shook his head.

"Oh, crap!" I stated.

"Gents. Let's finish our exam and roll him on his side so we can examine his back." The concern in my voice was unmistakable.

"One of you take the head, the other the feet, and I'll take the middle. Let's roll him together, gently, towards the door."

We all moved together and rolled him onto his left side. Dead center in the lower lumbar spine area was a dime-sized hole. It was not bleeding. The hole was below where the flak jacket would have ended if he was bending forward.

"OK, folks. Roll him toward me. Get an IV started now, and let's give him a dose of IV steroids. Nathan, step next door and tell them we're moving another patient to Immediate. Then get the front desk to call for a surgical Medevac for a spinal cord injury," I directed.

I turned to the patient to explain why he could not move his legs or feel his toes. He knew already from what we had said. His complete lack of pain was no longer reassuring. Off he went to the next room on the stretcher. Another medic carried the stretcher metal stands with him. The Immediate room was going to be more crowded.

The next bed held a gentleman in his late forties. He was in civilian clothes and was sitting up speaking loudly to the medic about his head and neck hurting.

"Hello, sir," I started as I grabbed an otoscope to look at his ears, pupils, and throat. "Let me look here," I said as I gazed in his left ear. "Oops, we don't seem to have an eardrum anymore on this side. Let me look in the other ear," I said as he turned toward me.

"Doc, my neck hurts," he repeated what I had overheard him tell the medic.

"Wow, I'm not surprised. Both your eardrums are gone. This is common in an IED explosion. The blast wave causes it," I observed.

"The good news is that the eardrums will grow back in a fairly short time," I added loudly as I continued his head, neck, heart and lung exams. All the rest seemed OK, so I reassured him and started to move to the next table.

"But, Doc, seriously, my neck is killing me," he pleaded. This made me pause. That was the third time he had said that. *Hmmm.*

I moved back to the table, touched his neck areas again, and said, "To make sure, let's get him a neck X-ray."

The medic nodded and led him around the corner, where we had a portable X-ray machine. It could display a digital image on our portable computer screen. I moved to the next table.

Five minutes later, the medic returned to say the X-ray was done. I sauntered over and looked at what was expected to display a normal neck. It was not normal.

"It seems like we did a good thing by getting his X-ray," I stated to all.

"Sir, your neck is broken. It looks like your C-4, fourth cervical vertebra, is broken into two pieces, and it's displaced badly. It's going to need surgery," I declared sympathetically.

"Please get this man a cervical soft collar," I directed the medic. After placing it securely, I advised him that he would be leaving soon on the next Medevac.

"Are you kidding me? I spent the last twenty years as an explosive ordnance Warrant Officer in the Marine Corps. Hell, I'm still on terminal leave with the Marines. So, you're telling me that on my first job as a civilian, with twenty years without an injury, I get here, get blown up, and have a broken neck?" he yelled.

"Yes, sir, Chief. Welcome to Iraq," I smiled.

Chapter 50 - Cut It Off!

I heard the stones and wood crash to the ground outside. Iraqi workers were restoring bombed-out huts to be used for lodging.

"Medic!" came the call from outside, and the two men closest to our main door grabbed their medical bags and rushed out.

One returned for a stretcher. A few minutes later, they both returned with a brown-dust-covered young man. His traditional Iraqi long white shirt, a dishdasha, was pulled up. The medics had exposed his left leg injury by cutting the leg of his loose-fitting cotton trousers. The two bones of his right lower leg were broken, the skin had scraped away, and the bones protruded from the wound. There was a small amount of active bleeding, and his leg was caked in desert dirt and clotted blood.

"Over here, please," I directed as they entered. We all moved to our emergency care area, and the canvas stretcher was placed in the middle. He was sixteen years old. He and his father had been working outside when a stone wall collapsed onto his son. They both spoke only a small amount of English, so we called over our interpreter.

It was a considerable wound involving much of the lateral aspect of his leg. The leg was bent at the break, twisted slightly, and two bones protruded from the wound. He was in pain.

"Get me ten milligrams of morphine, please," I directed.

"We will have to clean his wound and realign the leg. That will hurt a lot. Please ask if he is allergic to any medicines," I asked the interpreter. The father listened intently.

"No allergies," came the heavily accented reply from the father.

We gave the morphine and began to clean his leg with hydrogen peroxide and water rinses. The skin was mostly gone. Only a side flap remained. We used that to cover exposed muscle as best as we could.

Operational combat-area regulations stated that we could treat a local injury for anyone that came to our clinic. Once stable, an Iraqi national was to go to their local doctors for follow-on care. It seemed to me he would need antibiotics and an orthopedic surgeon to apply external fixators to hold the bones straight while they healed. This was a frequent and routinely successful procedure in the U.S.

Iraq was twenty-five years behind in medical knowledge under the Saddam Hussein regime, and external fixators were unheard of.

We had gently realigned his bones by pulling and letting his bone anatomy find its original positions. He moaned and groaned as we did it. His father gave him a rag to bite on.

"OK. We're done here," I announced. A sterile gauze bandage wrapped his entire lower leg.

"Let's get him in our ambulance and find out where his local clinic or hospital is," I finished, looking at the interpreter.

The dad and the boy listened as the interpreter explained the plan. Their eyes bulged wide and distress was in their voices.

"No, No! Cut off. Cut off!" said the father, as the boy nodded in agreement. The father was talking to the interpreter and making chopping motions with his hands above the boy's wound.

"Sir, the Iraqi doctors will amputate his leg," pronounced our helper.

I thought for a minute. "OK, got it. Let's call the gents next door and scramble a MedEvac bird up the road to our surgical hospital. There's an exception to the rule for locals to get our military care, and this is one of those exceptions," I commanded with authority.

Our MedEvac helicopters were conveniently stationed with us at the Habbaniya airfield. I sent a medic off to make the request in person. He would inform them that I had authorized the MedEvac and that we would follow immediately with our ambulance. Our patient and his father were hugging us and kissing our hands.

The helo took off noisily about thirty minutes later. We had called ahead to the surgical facility, ten minutes away by chopper, and told them what was coming. The orthopedic doctor there was a friend. Doctor Kelly Bal would do a superb job and save the boy's leg.

As the senior medical officer in the area and a 'full bird' colonel, I could requisition a helicopter any time I deemed it necessary.

The next morning, the clinic phone rang.

"Sir, there's a general on the line asking for you," stated the nervous medic at the front area.

"Colonel Adams, did you authorize a MedEvac yesterday for an Iraqi national with a broken leg?" he inquired.

"Yes, sir."

"Are you aware that Iraqis are not eligible for the use of our MedEvac and hospital facilities? They are supposed to be transferred to local care," he continued in a stern voice.

I had expected someone to call me about my decision. The one-star general calling himself was a shocker. He had overall command of our combat area and had a robust staff in support of area activities. I concluded that someone must have considered themselves imposed upon yesterday.

"Sir, as you know, we use all the resources at our disposal when we are treating 'life or limb' threatening injuries to locals. The young man had a compound fracture with bones exposed. He would have had his leg amputated if we had sent him to a local Iraqi facility. The Iraqi doctors are not capable of saving his leg, with his type of injury."

"Life or limb," I quoted from the regulations.

"Roger that, Doc, and I appreciate your explanation," he paused, then concluded, "And the prompt actions by all. Carry on."

I could tell he was happier than when he first called.

Chapter 51 – Midnight Ambulance Transfer – Pediatric Hero

I slept in the on-call room dressed in my dirty uniform and covered with a light blanket to keep the sand-flies from munching on me all night. It was 2 AM.

"Sir, there's a call for you from headquarters about a casualty coming in," stated the wide-awake medic. I shook the cobwebs away and moved to the one clinic field phone.

"Doctor Adams. This is not a secure line," I answered.

The news was disconcerting. Because of rare rain in the desert, helicopters were grounded. An Iraqi combatant had tried to drive his bomb-loaded truck past the Division headquarters gate two hours away. American bullets riddled him and his truck, but the truck did not detonate. He was alive with multiple gunshot wounds, a right arm partial amputation with a tourniquet in place and was coming to our location by ground ambulance.

We were not a surgery center. That was located a long three hours away by ambulance. Our job was to do an ambulance transfer. We would need to stabilize him for the follow-on trip. The ambulance bringing him to us would return to headquarters following regulations that did not allow it to make the more extended trip.

I called for one other doctor and two medics from our barracks a mile away. What arrived were all three animated doctors and more medics. The headquarters ambulance arrived forty-five minutes later in a light drizzle.

"Bring him here please," directed Doctor Conlan, who now oversaw triage. The medics carried the stretcher to our mobile stand in the Immediate room and placed the stretcher down. The patient moaned.

"He has a ninety percent right arm partial amputation with a tourniquet in place and holding," Mary began for all to hear.

"There are three bullet wounds in the chest and abdomen, and only one exit wound in the back near the right buttocks," she continued as the exam progressed.

"There's an old subclavian central line, and a left femoral IV in place. Neither one is functioning, and IV fluid is not running in," she continued. He moaned again as she rolled him flat.

"Has he been given any pain meds?" she asked the medic with the transfer paperwork.

"He was given ten milligrams of morphine a little over two hours ago in Ramadi," he replied.

"OK," she said and glanced over at me. "Let's give him ten more of morphine now," she stated with a question in her eyes. I nodded.

"Give it in his buttock, please. His IV isn't working, and we need IV access," she directed.

The medic was trying to start a new IV line. He replied he could not find a vein or much of a pulse.

"Doctor Dobson. Time for your magic, please. If you can get an IV in a newborn baby's scalp, you should be able to get an IV started somewhere," I stated encouragingly. He was a pediatrician.

He moved his athletic five-foot nine-inch frame to the table and reached for a small 23-gauge butterfly needle. He stretched out the long, small bore, transparent tubing attached and went to work. After a few attempts at the left arm and both feet, he claimed defeat.

"I can't see or feel the veins to get a needle in. He has lost too much blood," he stated with concern.

I had been going through the ATLS (Advanced Trauma Life Support) course in my head and decided to try something I had only done on animal patients before.

"Go to the call room please, and bring me the ATLS manual, on the first shelf next to the bed," I requested to the medic nearest me.

"We are going to try a venous ankle cut-down."

I found the page I needed, opened the book, and placed it between the legs of our patient. "There's a large foot vein that runs behind the medial ankle bone." I began to instruct as I went.

"I will make a cut in the skin here, above the medial malleolus, and dissect down until we find the large saphenous vein." I made the cut precisely, and the patient moaned again. The medic dabbed away a small amount of blood and redirected the surgical light to the wound area.

"Look. There it is," I pointed with the scalpel. "It's right next to a small nerve. I am going to lift it up so you can get a suture under it," I directed. The medic helped in awe.

We ran the suture under the pale vein, and I made a small nick in the surface of the vein. This allowed us to thread a large-bore IV catheter into the vein. I tied it in place with the sutures, rolled the skin back in place, and reached for the IV bag control device. It started to flow rapidly, and the room erupted in applause. I received high fives from Doctor Dobson and my medic.

"Wow. That was the first time I've done that on a human," I noted, pretty proud of myself.

"Let's use this access to give him ten more milligrams of morphine and get him into our ambulance. We need a medic to go on the transfer," I finished.

Ten minutes later, Doctor Dobson was in the ambulance with the young medic showing him how to draw up the correct dose of morphine from a larger vial. The medic was concentrating.

"OK, Doc, come on out. We need to get the show going. They've got a three-hour ride ahead, through bad guy country," I stated. The only light was from the red glow inside the ambulance. Darkness surrounded us. He and I both knew regulations stated that doctors do not go on ambulance transfers. It is too risky. Doctors were in short supply, so it was the medic's job.

"Sir, I need to go," he stated with a pleading expression.

"Craig, you know the rules. I need you here," I stated sympathetically.

He repeated it with a concerned emphasis that got my attention. "Sir, I need to go." I thought about it and knew he and I would both be taking a risk if I let him do this.

I made a command decision based on permission from our battalion commander that allowed us to go with our gut feelings. He was not telling me something.

"OK, Craig, you can go. But you get the first helo back here in the morning. Promise?"

"Yes, sir," he replied with relief in his voice. His dark brown eyes were steady and determined as he returned to the task of keeping the patient alive.

He returned the next morning by hitching a 3.5 hour ride back on the returning Division armed convoy.

He came to report in and thank me for letting him go.

"Welcome back. What was that all about last night? You put me in a tough spot."

"Bob, that medic you sent with me was scared to death. I could not get him to understand simple instructions about giving the pain meds. I was almost sure our patient would die during the trip, and I did not want that on his conscience. His death needed to be my responsibility alone."

I was taken aback by this. His risky request and my rule-breaking decision had happened because he wanted to protect the future psychologic health of our medic.

I regret to this day that I did not put him in for a medal for his act of compassion and heroism. I did make sure, years later, that he knew of my deep respect for his character and the decision he made that night.

Commentary: Everyone in the room was angry at the man who had tried to kill our fellow teammates. We did not care about his pain as much as we would if it had been one of our own. But there was no question in anyone's mind that our primary responsibility was to save lives. There was a common understanding that this casualty had wanted to die to take as many of *his enemy* with him as he could.

We wanted to let him live.

That was what they trained us for, and that was what we did. We hoped that one day his children might live in a peaceful world.

And: *Colonel* Dobson added the following after reading this chapter.

"The route of the convoy was an interesting detail. Fallujah was in enemy hands. It was not taken until April 2004. We went to our battalion commander and explained that the casualty wouldn't survive the 3.5-hour route around Fallujah, but if we used the *black* (off-limits) route of the highway through town, it would cut the time to less than an hour. The decision was made to take the faster route because in the horrible weather (sand/rainstorm) and at night, the enemy would never suspect a U.S. convoy blowing through town.

The convoy commander came to me and asked, *Doc, how fast can we drive with your casualty?*

Fast as hell, Sergeant. Just don't wreck."

They did precisely that, and the patient lived. *My hero.*

Chapter 52 – Steroid Rash and Infectious Diseases

Iraq is a hot, desolate, light-brown desert land that is host to hordes of biting insects. Sand-flies and sand fleas were everywhere, and they were the same color as the sand and barely visible. Mosquito nets were essential to sleep, but not always available or effective. Patients were coming to our clinic covered head-to-toe with bug bites. There was a slight difference between the fly bites -- that carried the risk of Leishmaniasis diseases and flea bites -- which itched more. I had been trying to show my medics and staff how to tell the difference.

"Colonel, can you come see the rash we're looking at? We can't tell if these are flea or fly bites," requested the medic.

I followed him to a cot where a young female Army Captain sat. I took a careful look at her face, back, arms, and upper chest. These were not bug bites. I was looking at something different, and I noticed she was muscular and had the shadow of well-shaved chin hair.

"How long have you been using steroids?" I started.

"I don't use steroids, sir," she responded in a deep, almost male voice.

I noticed her West Point ring.

"You have large muscles and small breasts," I countered. "This rash of yours looks like the rash that bodybuilders get when they are using steroids. So, Captain, on your honor as a West Point grad, are you using steroids?" I tested again.

"Absolutely not, sir," she responded promptly. "I was a three-sport athlete at West Point, and I've gone to other doctors about this rash in the past. They told me it was acne, but their treatments didn't work. I came here hoping you might have a better answer," she concluded in a husky voice.

Now she had my attention. "Do you, by any chance, like salt?" I queried.

Her eyes got wide, and she said emphatically, "I crave the stuff."

This was a clue to her previously missed diagnosis. I turned to the medic and asked him to get a urine sample to look at her sodium level. He led her to our makeshift lab and gave her a urine cup. After he had dipped it, he came to me with the results.

"Sir, her sodium level is very low, and her specific gravity is abnormal. Is that helpful?"

"Yes, it is." We moved back to her cot, and I began my mini-lecture for her and the medics.

"Captain, you don't have acne. These are not bug bites, as you already knew. This is a rash frequently caused by the use of steroids. But, since you have never used steroids, we must ask ourselves why you have all the same signs. Your deep voice, chin hair, athletic, muscular build, and small breasts all point to steroids in your system. The explanation is that you have an adrenal gland that is overproducing steroids," I lectured.

"It's most likely from a tumor in the mineralocorticoid layer of one of your adrenal glands. That is why you crave salt, and your urine shows you're low in sodium. I'm surprised it was not found years ago, but it may simply be getting worse now," I concluded, pleased with diagnosing a rare disorder in the war-torn desert of a foreign country.

"The good news is it's certainly a benign tumor, or you would have been dead by now. So, as of now, you can eat all the salt you want," I concluded.

"Thank you, sir, I will absolutely do that. I had been avoiding it. But what do I do now?" she finished with concern in her voice.

"We could MedEvac you home for further evaluation if you want. But you've had it for some time. It will eventually need surgery, but you can safely finish your tour here and get it fixed when you get back. What would you like to do?"

"I would like to eat salt and finish my tour, sir. Thank you very much. This answers a lot of questions for me," she said, smiling.

She left. The medics were impressed.

Dang, I love the practice of medicine.

Chapter 53 - Diseases in the Sand

Leishmaniasis is an infectious disease carried by sand-flies, and sand-flies were everywhere. They feasted on us at night. Wild dogs were carriers since the flies bit them too. Since the war began, cats and dogs had flourished. There was no longer any Iraqi animal control since the collapse of government operations.

I was ordered to explore ways to keep dogs away from our operational area. It was medically appropriate. I found some enlisted hunters to help me track and shoot wild dogs coming to eat our trash. If a hunt were successful, we would move the dead dogs to the road and call for a disposal truck to pick them up and move them to a burn area. We were often unsuccessful. The dogs were clever at avoiding contact.

I returned from one hunting outing to find Doctor Mary Conlan and a female medic behind our clinic building, giving water to an injured dog.

"What are you doing?" I demanded softly.

"This poor dog has had puppies, and she's hurt," they responded in concerned voices.

"Can't we help her? Maybe she can become a unit pet," finished Doctor Conlan.

"Ladies. Please go back inside. I will take care of this," I stated in my best command voice.

"What? What are you going to do?" she responded with alarm.

"I'm going to do my job. Please go inside."

I waited until I was alone. The dog was panting and lying on her side, watching me.

I drew my issue 9 mm pistol, charged it, and fired at close range. It was a difficult thing to do, but another option was not viable. The animal was infected and posed a risk to others. I moved the carcass to the road edge, went inside, and asked the medic to call for a disposal van.

Mary did not speak to me for several days, which I totally understood.

A large, cool, spring-fed lake bordered one edge of our encampment area. We had established a guarded swim area that allowed hot soldiers to swim at the end of long, dry, exhausting days. It was a godsend. But it did not last long.

The rivers feeding into the lake contained snails that were infected with schistosomiasis parasites. There were three types of these parasites. Some infected human skin and caused visible sores, while others were more dangerous and invaded the veins and internal organs. Dogs, cats, and rodents were carriers. They were infected by wading in and drinking the water the snails lived in.

These waterborne parasites could also infect humans. The immature parasite in water could swim up the human urethra into the bladder, and then on to other organs. Once the senior general discovered this fact, the swim area was closed. I tried to save it by pointing out that schistosomiasis was rare and treatable. It was in the same family as pinworms that all our children are exposed to in kindergarten. No luck.

After the lake closed to swimming, a female presented to our clinic with urinary tract symptoms.

"Have you been swimming in our lake?" I asked after taking a detailed history for urinary infections.

"Yes, many times. I miss it," she responded.

I grabbed the medic. "Let's go check her urine. We have a centrifuge. We can spin the urine and look for schistosomiasis eggs," I directed. "They are quite large under a microscope and look similar to the pinworm eggs I've seen in my children when they were young."

We prepared a microscope slide with her centrifuge-spun urine.

"Look here," I started triumphantly, pointing to the microscope. "Those are eggs. She's got schistosomiasis. Our first confirmed case," I concluded. It was easy to treat. One pill of a standard 'anthelmintic' drug would cure her. Unfortunately, we did not have any.

Our supply system was robust after the first few months in-country, so I ordered a bottle of the needed drug, and a week later, our patient returned for her one pill treatment. One week after that, she was symptom-free, and her urine was back to normal.

I would later develop a lesion on my chin that was diagnosed as cutaneous leishmaniasis. I took one of the same medicines for this new schistosomiasis. My thought was I could treat both my past lake swimming risk and this new bug-bite related sore with the same drug. That was not supported by literature, but I had other worries in a war zone.

The chin lesion went away after a month and did not return.

Chapter 54 – Will You Deliver My Baby?

I received a call from Baghdad. The senior doctor in that operational area, also a colonel, wanted me to move there to take over a USAID humanitarian operation that could change the face of medicine in Iraq. They had a USAID $250,000 grant and a plan. I was asked to help make it a reality. We were authorized to conduct a conference for Iraqi physicians detailing advances in medical and surgical care over the last three decades.

Saddam Hussein had forbidden the Internet, outside television, and travel by doctors. We were also encouraged to introduce the concept of a medical organization to this newly emerging democratic country.

A week later, I was on a helo to Baghdad with most of my personal possessions. I was given an office in the now-occupied enormous palace of Saddam Hussein. Huge bronze heads of 'Saddam the Warrior' graced the four corner roofs. They were being removed by large cranes when I arrived.

There was an active clinic next to my office where a physician assistant and I could also see patients.

Soon after setting up business in the palace, I was asked to consider helping an American in need. She was a lovely, young, and pregnant lady. Her sparkling brown eyes, auburn hair, and a perfect smile captivated me. She had not known she was pregnant when she had accepted the most important job of her life. She was working downtown helping to rebuild the war-ravaged countryside. USAID provided the rebuilding tools. Her name was Nobel, and her actions suggested her name had a special meaning. She was six months pregnant, and we were at war.

"Everyone has already told me to go back to the states," she stated evenly, with pleading eyes. "I am not going back. The nuns downtown are willing to deliver me, but they don't even have electricity. I sincerely thank you for seeing me today," she stated.

"I agree you should go back, but if you won't, I would hate to see you forced to go to the nuns. One problem, as you know, is that as an employee of USAID, you're not eligible for military care. Nonetheless, I can follow you in my clinic here, and I believe I can convince our hospital commander that we can consider your situation both unique and worthy of an exception. I'll ask her today and let you know," I said sincerely.

"Thank you, Doctor. I really, really appreciate your help," she exclaimed, smiling, with tears in her glowing brown eyes.

"Absolutely not!" came the reply to my carefully worded request for permission to deliver the baby in our local hospital. The military had taken over Iraq's ex-president Saddam Hussein's large and modern medical facility and converted it into an emergency casualty center and hospital. It was now equipped with our modern surgical and medical equipment.

"We can't accept that kind of liability. I'm an OB/GYN doctor, and I would not dream of letting her have her baby here. It's not safe or right. We don't have a pediatrician or neonatologist here if the baby has problems," she stated quite forcefully.

We were both doctors and colonels. We were in her private office and dressed in desert camouflage as a visual reminder of where we were. I would not win the argument with rank or logic, but I tried.

"You're also a woman, and she's an American," I concluded. "We have the ability to help. You can't actually want local Iraqi nuns to deliver her in a facility without electricity?"

"Not in my hospital," was her final statement on the subject.

I thanked her for her time and left both angry and disappointed. *We are at war. Liability would not be a concern when helping an American in need in a war zone.*

OB/GYN doctors are the most sued specialty. I understood her concern based on the life she led back home. This, nonetheless, was not a place where malpractice lawyers spent any time at all.

After a moment weighing my options, I made my way across the street to the presidential palace. The area 'Green Zone' commander was a British 2-star general. He had a solid reputation as a military leader.

"Sir," I started after saluting, "I appreciate your time. There's an important matter I need your help with."

"Right mate," he responded with a thick British accent, as he leaned back to hear more.

I explained the situation from the beginning, where I had been approached to help and further acknowledged regulations making her ineligible for our military medical care.

"The simple problem here, sir, is that the USAID agency in Baghdad does not have any medical ability to deliver a baby. The nuns that deliver local babies sometimes don't have electricity in their bombed and damaged convent. She wants to stay here, knowing the risks because she knows that what she's doing here, helping the local population, is the most important job she's ever had."

"I'm asking you to consider the unique nature of the situation. I want to deliver this American baby safely here in our very capable facility. The commander is an obstetrician, and available if needed, but she's refusing my use of the facility," I stated, with a concerned but professional tone.

"My question, sir, is, can you make an exception to policy in this case, or do you want me to send her downtown to the nuns?"

He leaned back in his chair, in reflection.

In his best, extremely British, deep command voice, he responded, "Oh right, mate. Like there's more than one answer to that question?" And he smiled.

Three months later, we delivered a beautiful baby girl in our hospital. A neonatologist had been found in a unit nearby and flown in by the now cooperative hospital commander. His unique skills were not needed as it turned out, but we all enjoyed this moment of joy in a bad place.

She named her little girl Allie and sent me pictures of her for many years so we could both enjoy watching her grow up.

Chapter 55 – Iraqi Medical Specialty Forum

The Army command in Habbaniya sent me a medic and a Medical Service Corps officer to staff the project I was helping with. I had requested someone who could type well, and Specialist Serena Hare had won the typing contest for applicants. CPT Aaron Anderson was a Medical Service Officer that I had requested by name. His administrative skills were well known to me. He came with her on the helo that flew them to Baghdad with all their personal effects.

Our mission was to arrange a conference for Iraqi physicians to update them on the changes in medicine across all specialties that had occurred in the last twenty-five years. The capable and dedicated Iraq physicians practiced the same way they did twenty-five years ago. Progress had stopped.

It was dangerous to leave the secure embassy area Green Zone, but we needed to pick up our $250,000 in cash from the USAID compound in downtown Baghdad. There were no operating banks after the initial invasion, so the money was in cash, stuffed in a backpack.

The three of us changed into civilian clothes, added bulletproof vests under our jackets, and climbed into the back of a small local pickup truck driven by an Iraqi doctor. This ex-military doctor had been a 2-star general and Assistant Surgeon General of Iraq. Since our invading force had disbanded the military, he now gratefully worked for us.

"Bring your weapons, and keep them visible," I started my briefing. "In case we're followed or encounter anyone suspicious, show your weapons, and look like you will use them. Bring extra magazines but pray we won't need them. The trip to the USAID offices should be short," I concluded.

The traffic was just plain stupid. There were no working stoplights and no police. Traffic moved in both directions on both sides of the roads. Traffic circles had cars choosing the easiest path, and we found cars traveling around them in both directions.

"What do you do if there's an accident? You don't have insurance, do you?" I wondered out loud after our physician driver swerved again to slip around another pile of disconnected drivers.

"We get out and inspect the damage. If we can still drive, we say *inshallah,* and move on," he replied logically.

Inshallah is a beautiful word, and it is used often. It means 'God willing, or if God wills.' When I said 'goodbye, I will see you tomorrow,' the response was often, *inshallah* – if God wills. I loved that response.

The trip back was nerve-wracking. We rode in an old rickety pickup truck with the cash-stuffed backpack tucked between the medic's legs on the passenger side. Her blond hair was in a ponytail, and her AK-47 was loaded and visible. Another passenger, CPT Anderson sat in the open back leaning against the cab window. He carried a 9 mm officer's pistol under his jacket and kept his hand on it while staring directly at the driver of any car that followed. Everyone wore bulletproof vests under our jackets. We traveled as fast as was safe and made it back without a problem. *Whew.*

Our small staff worked long days to plan a four-day conference and arrange to fly thirty-two physicians across multiple specialties to Iraq in 2004. Active fighting continued. We would fly them into Jordan, where a military transport plane would fly them to Baghdad.

We spent a lot of our funds on upgrading a conference facility in the downtown area. Because of security concerns, it would be challenging to allow hundreds of doctors from all over Iraq to enter the more secure Green Zone for a four-day conference. We were advertising the conference on the newly working Internet. Satellite dishes were popping up on rooftops all over Iraq. Cell phone networks were being established, and modern communications blossomed.

The American and British doctors were en route to Jordan when I received a letter from an Iraqi doctor. His letter indicated, in no uncertain terms, that our conference would be a target for a bombing. He wrote that members of his own family were part of the plot. He had been planning to attend when he learned of the planned attack on his countrymen, physicians, and women.

The conference was scheduled to begin in three days. We had U.S. sniper and security forces arranged, and the downtown Baghdad facility had been repaired at significant cost, with new lighting and plumbing. It was a showpiece now.

"Sir, we have a problem," I declared to the British two-star general in charge of the area.

"This letter states that we need to cancel the upcoming Iraqi Medical Specialty Forum conference because of a credible threat that we will be a bombing target. As I see it, sir, we have two choices. We can cancel the conference and send all the doctors home from Jordan, where they are now. Or we can move the conference from downtown to inside the protected Green Zone," I concluded.

"Sir, honestly, what we're going to do with the conference will change the face of medicine in this country overnight. We're planning to jump-start Iraq into the modern world of current medical practice in just four days."

"What would you need to do this, Doc?" he asked suspiciously. I could see his thoughts spinning.

I had already discussed this with our Iraqi ex-Surgeon General and my staff.

"We would need the use of the Green Zone conference center, and we would need enough buses to transport 500 physicians from the planned site to and from our conference center each day for four days. We would need a company of Marines to conduct the search, screening, and transportation process. And there are several activities currently planned at the conference center. Many of them would have to be relocated or rescheduled," I summarized.

His operations officer was present in the room. The general turned to him.

"Do we have the buses and Marines the doc needs for the planned four days?"

"Yes sir, I can make that happen," came the surprising but welcome response.

"Well, Doc, we have spent a lot of money so far. Why don't you get with Operations and make it happen?" he smiled. And so, did I.

It worked. We pulled off a bait-and-switch operation. The 500 doctors showed up where and when we had advertised. We loaded them onto the waiting buses, issued I.D. badges, searched each attendee, and escorted them into the Green Zone. Marines provided security the whole way.

The event was a resounding success. The Surgeon General of the Army flew in as our opening guest speaker, and for four days we taught doctors about medical progress over the last three decades.

Iraqi doctors came to us in tears. "We never dreamed something like this would happen in our country in our lifetimes," they sobbed.

"God bless America, and thank you for our new freedoms," they often concluded. We were stunned and honored.

On the first day of our planned event, bomb-sniffing dogs found the large explosive cache placed in the original conference center. It was disarmed and removed without incident.

We made a CD-ROM of the lectures given by each visiting physician and presented one of them to each attendee. Multiple specialties were represented. Within a month of the conference's end, over 5,000 copies were made by the attendees and were circulating in Iraqi medical facilities all over the country.

Iraq had been recognized for the most capable medical resources in the Middle East years before, and it is rapidly becoming the best again.

When our medical unit in Habbaniya was ready to rotate home, the 82nd Airborne headquarters called the three of us in Baghdad and asked if we could be ready in two days to return home with them on their scheduled aircraft. We were officially assigned to the 82nd.

Our response was energetic. We were packed and back by helo the next day. I had paused at the Baghdad commander's office first and asked for a commendation medal for my two staff.

He responded in a wonderfully British way. "Oh, right mate. You Americans like medals. We just like to say, *Good job, mate. March on.* I'll take care of it, and I'm going to throw one in for you too." He called his chief of staff to the office, and the award forms were completed in minutes. It's good to be a general.

The C-130 transport aircraft did not stop as it slowly turned on the Habbaniya runway to line up for takeoff. Stopping the plane would make it an easy target for mortars. Our entire unit lined up, heavy bags in our hands, and watched the rear door ramp open as the plane turned. We moved in single file, dragging our gear, and climbed up the grey rear metal ramp. None of us had ever boarded a moving aircraft before, but in a war zone, much of what we did was new.

Chapter 56 - Going Home

As a full bird colonel in a war zone, I was informed that my way home could be made easier if I wished. The current travel plan was to fly from Habbaniya, Iraq, to the Ballad, Iraq airbase, spend the night there and catch a plane to Turkey. From Turkey, we would wait for transport to Frankfurt, Germany, and from there await a ride home to Fort Bragg, NC. The whole process could take seven to ten days.

On arrival in Ballad, I was invited to register for a space available seat on one of four planes expected that day going directly to Frankfurt, Germany. I offloaded my bags, bid farewell to my medics and staff, and settled down in the airport waiting area alone.

The third plane out that night had room for one more passenger and I made the list. It was a last-minute decision by the pilot, and I was rushed through the military customs area as a VIP. The customs process was quick and cursory.

The aircraft was a vast C-141 Strategic Airlifter Transport. The crew loaded it front-to-back with military vehicles tied to the floor. Along the sides were pull-down web seats for passengers. I found an empty space and settled in with the others for a five-hour flight.

I was taken aback on landing when a Staff Sergeant climbed on board and called my name.

"Colonel Adams, can you show me which bags are yours, sir? We have a vehicle outside for you," he observed respectfully.

In the vehicle was an Army Major as a driver. This was special treatment due to my rank that both pleased and astonished me.

"Sir, do you have any civilian clothes?" queried the Major when we arrived in the VIP lounge at the Frankfurt airport.

"I have one set in the bottom of my duffel," I replied.

"Well, put those on, sir. There's a shower over there. Take a nap, and we will be back to get you in about five hours. We have you booked on a Delta Airlines flight in the morning," he smiled, knowing I was a bit surprised.

Five hours later, they arrived and escorted me to the Delta Airlines commercial waiting area. They checked my bags for me, handed me my tickets, and wished me well.

I had the desert camouflage shoulder backpack that had come with my standard-issue Molle II Standard Pack system. It contained a shaving kit, food, and clean underwear.

I moved toward the security screening area with anticipation. There was an airport duty-free store past the checkpoint, and I was contemplating picking up some cheap liquor to take home with me. It had been six months since I had even sniffed a beer.

I threw my backpack on the conveyor belt and moved along with the line of people in front of me. I was enjoying myself.

"Sir, can you take a look at this, and tell me what you have in your pack side pocket?" demanded the German screener. He wore a military uniform.

I glanced at the X-ray display and saw what he was pointing to.

"I'm not sure what that is. I think maybe - batteries?" I stated with doubt in my voice.

"I don't think so, sir. I am going to call my supervisor."

A uniformed and alert female German officer showed up. She had a sidearm on her waist and was carrying a shoulder-slung MP-5 submachine gun.

"Sir, would you please remove the contents of that pocket?" she ordered as she unslung her MP-5 into a ready position.

I reached into the pocket and grabbed a cardboard box. I knew what it was immediately, and I realized I was in a lot of deep doo-doo. I pulled out a fresh box of standard U.S. issue 9mm pistol ammunition.

I thought with alarm about how to get out of this apparent international jam.

"Ma'am, I don't need these anymore. And they work well in the MP-5 you are carrying," I said sincerely, and smiling. I held the box out toward her.

"That would make my paperwork much easier," she stated in a commanding voice with her hand outstretched. I handed the box of bullets to her and waited.

She nodded to the screener, winked at me, and turned away with her new package. We were on the same team, after all.

I had waited to call my wife until I had cleared the screener and heard my flight being called. I did not want a travel delay disappointment. It would be devastating after so long.

"Sweetheart, I will be home tonight on Delta airlines. Please pick me up at the Fayetteville airport," I said into the public wall-phone receiver.

She giggled loudly with surprise and delight.

I settled into a row of empty seats up front, and the flight attendant brought a cart with beer, wine, and liquor to my row.

"I expect it may have been a long time since anyone asked you this but would you like an alcoholic beverage?" she smiled. "It's on me."

I had a beer. It was delicious.

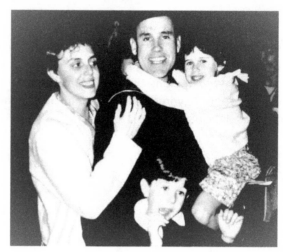

Graduation at Wake Forest University Medical School 1991

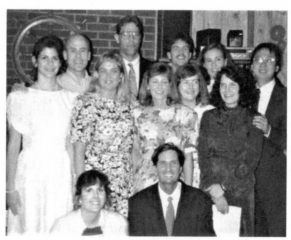

Wake Forest University Medical School's
first Parallel Curriculum class

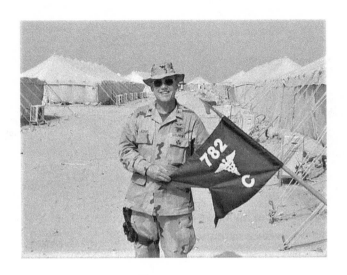

Deployment with the 82nd Airborne Division 782nd Medical Company came to Iraq via Kuwait

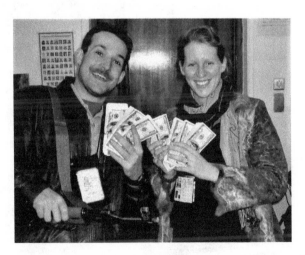

Soldiers Aaron Anderson and Serena Hare with $250,000 cash in Iraq for the USAID grant – no banks were functioning in 2004

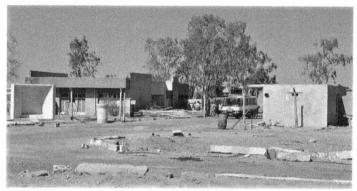

Habbaniya, Iraq buildings on an abandoned airfield that we turned
into a full-service medical facility in 2003

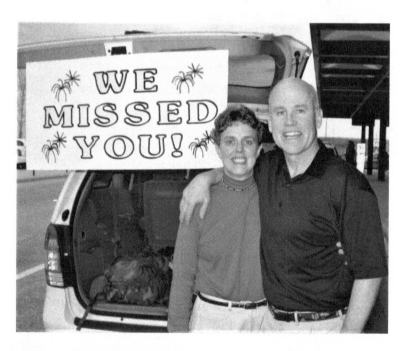

Homecoming in Fayetteville, NC. Back from Iraq in 2004

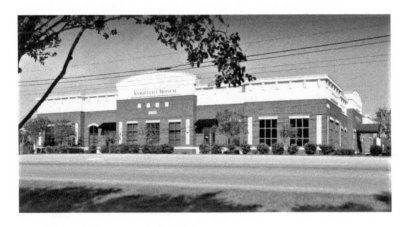

Knightdale Family Medicine in my 14,000 square foot multi-specialty medical building

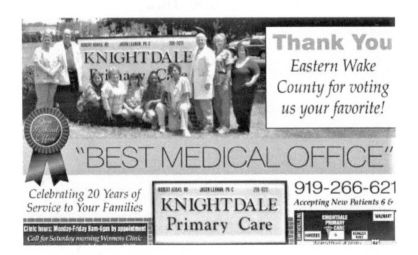

Our first Knightdale clinic won Best Medical Clinic Awards 2007, 2008 and 2009

"The art of medicine is to be properly learned only from its practice and its exercise."
Thomas Sydenham

PRIVATE PRACTICE

Chapter 57 – Tetany in a Soldier

He was twenty-six years old and the finest physical specimen of a fit male I had ever seen. His muscles were defined and taught. He was handsome and alert, with intelligent eyes, and his hair was cut short in a military style.

"I feel like crap, Doc," he started as we shook hands. He knew I had a military background and had asked to see me as a new patient in the private practice I had joined after retiring from the military the month before.

I smiled and admired his direct approach. His fiancée looked on with interest, but not worry.

"I understand you have just returned from Afghanistan," I noted. "What did you do there?"

"I was a sniper up in the mountains. We moved around a lot. I got back last week for some R&R for three weeks. I go back to finish my tour in two weeks, but I have not been feeling well since I got home. Food tastes bland, and I have a headache every day. I rarely get headaches unless I drink too much," he smiled weakly.

"OK, let's look at you. Take off clothes to your underwear, and we will check. Do you want your girlfriend to stay?"

"Yes, please. She's the one who insisted I get a checkup," he smiled. She did not.

I conducted a complete neurologic exam, peered at his eyes and retina with my ophthalmoscope, and finished a comprehensive physical exam, but skipped the testicle and rectal exam.

I noticed with admiration how very fit he appeared. His muscles were defined and firm. His vital signs were normal, and he had the low blood pressure of an athlete, with a resting heart rate of 50.

I was stumped, but only slightly concerned. He had been eating field rations, wandering the high-altitude mountains, and sleeping on dirt and rocks. Now he was eating McDonald's and drinking beer.

"I'll be honest with you both. There's nothing obvious I can find to explain why you feel bad. I'm going to need to do lab work to see if I can get a clue as to why you feel this way," I stated. I ordered all the labs I could think of, including a thyroid panel and a sedimentation rate. The sedimentation rate is a measure of inflammation and can suggest infection, cancer, or autoimmune issues.

"The nurse will take you to the lab, and I'll call you with the results tomorrow. Please make an appointment for next week before you leave so that we can review things again."

It was a Friday, and I moved on to my next patient.

Saturday began with a check of patients in the hospital. I was on call for the weekend for the practice. At 9 AM, I had checked on the two inpatients, wrote notes in their charts, and pulled up my labs for review. All the labs from yesterday were available.

There were three sets of labs I had not seen. One was from my mystery soldier seen the day before.

All the labs were perfect except for the sedimentation rate. It was quite elevated. All I had now was more confusion. *Cancer? Infection? Autoimmune?* The other labs should have shown some abnormality if any of those diagnoses were correct.

I went home and ate breakfast. Something was wrong, but I could not see it. I went over the physical exam in my head again -- top to bottom. All that stood out was how fit he was. His abdominal muscles were as tight as a washboard, which I admired.

"Wait." They were tight. *What's the medical word for tight muscles? Tetany. Oh, no. He could have tetanus!* He had been crawling on his hands and knees in the dirt of Afghanistan, where the locals would piss and defecate outside. Germs were everywhere.

"This is Doctor Adams at the Med One clinic, sir," I stated when the hospital CEO answered his cell phone. It was Saturday morning. "I have been asked to call you in order for you to release the tetanus anti-toxin shot you have in stock. It's your only one in stock."

"Doctor, we keep that shot on hand for a tetanus emergency. We have not had a case here recently that I can remember. Why do you need it?" he inquired doubtfully.

"Sir, I have an Army soldier recently returned from Afghanistan with an exam and labs suspicious for tetanus. He's high risk and currently sick. I'll order the confirmation test on Monday, but I have directed him to come back from out of town today, so I can give him this shot, and save his life."

There was silence for a few seconds. I was speaking to an administrator, not a physician, but he made the right call.

"I will direct the pharmacy to release the shot to you, Doctor. I would like you to copy me on the confirmation lab next week. If positive, we'll report it to our health department."

The soldier and his girlfriend arrived back in town from her parent's house that afternoon. I opened the office so we could give the shot and draw blood to confirm infection by the tetanus bacterium Clostridium tetani.

I administered the vaccine, and they were counseled on symptoms that would require them to call or come back. They were grateful and concerned. The test results came back on Monday afternoon, and I sent a copy by email to the CEO with thanks. It was positive for Clostridium tetani.

Whew.

Chapter 58 – First Civilian Clinic – Big Mistake?

Military medicine is unique in several ways. The benefits included free care to my patients and the absence of lawyers or insurance companies influencing providers on how to practice. Medicine was free, and the prescriptions that were written got filled. In the civilian world, a considerable percentage of prescriptions go unfilled, primarily due to cost.

There are no military malpractice insurance policies or similar costs to practice in uniform. The U.S. government is the insurer.

When I stepped out of uniform to begin private practice, I could no longer deliver babies or do vasectomies for my patients. The cost of malpractice insurance was too high to allow me to do what I had done for years.

I would now care for illnesses that were rare in my past. Diabetes and drug abuse ran rampant in my new patient population. The military had weight standards, so diabetes was unusual, even in families. Annual military drug screening was a useful tool to limit the drug use problem.

When I got a letter offering me a job in Knightdale, NC, near where my son lived, I showed it to Jeri, and we agreed to check it out. I had already started a new civilian job with a large family medicine group as the junior doctor but had a hard time dealing with the organization that cared little about my past experiences.

The Knightdale clinic, which I visited to evaluate for a future job, was unique. It had five exam rooms and needed an MD to supervise the one current physician assistant. The administrative and nursing staffs were experienced and capable, and the small community had never had a full-service family physician. I studied the financial information, saw it had good potential, and rushed home to suggest we take the job.

My willing wife agreed. We put the house on the market, and I moved to neighboring Raleigh to start a job where I would be the boss again. In all my posts with the Army, I had been the chief. There were always superior officers to deal with, but at my clinics, I was the boss. This was a job I understood and thrived in.

I was excited about the opportunity and was quickly busy. The clinic was popular with the community, and word got out rapidly that there was a new full-service doctor in town.

Four days later, I called Jeri in distress.

"Sweetheart, I have made a huge mistake. This place is an absolute disaster. A large portion of the patients are coming in for narcotic drug refills, the staff seems unhappy most of the time, and angry patients are yelling at my staff when I suggest they stop using drugs," I summarized unhappily.

"Honestly?" she asked. "You know you signed a three-year contract, don't you?" she responded. "I'm down here packing up and selling our house. So, let me ask you a couple of questions. How many clinics did you command in the Army?"

"Five," I responded quickly.

"How many of those clinics were disasters when you took them over?" she continued.

"Five," I responded, knowing where she was going.

"And how many of those won awards for excellence within a year of you taking over?"

"Five," I concluded, knowing now what she would say next.

"Well, then, shut up and fix it. I have a house to move," she concluded lovingly.

I started the next day the same way I had started in all my past attempts. I gathered the staff and asked if they were happy. They were not.

I told them I wanted us to be the best full-service family clinic in the state and would allow each of them to do whatever they needed to do to make that happen. It enabled them.

"Let's make some changes. I'll give our drug users help to quit using, or we will ask them to find another clinic. We will take care of our patients, as a family, and take care of ourselves equally well," I concluded. The change began that day, and it was a different place. We were a team on a mission to create an environment where we could be proud and happy.

Sixty percent of our drug-addicted patients worked with us and became gratefully drug-free. The rest went away, reminding us that it would not be difficult for them to find a doctor to give them what they wanted. Unfortunately, that was true. Fortunately, they would now become someone else's problem patient.

We sold the house, moved to Raleigh, and started our new life.

Eleven months later, our clinic was featured in the local paper. The paper had done a "Best of Everything" reader survey.

A reporter came by to ask us who we were. "We have never heard of you," began the reporter.
"You won all the votes for Best Medical Clinic across all the many specialties. Who are you guys?"
   We smiled and let them take out picture. We were happy again.

Chapter 59 – God Did It

1 Peter 4:10 – "Each of you should use whatever gift you have received to serve others, as faithful stewards of God's grace in its various forms."

A year after we had started our new clinic, as a team focused on our patients and not ourselves, my head nurse found me. It was lunchtime.

"I'm going to visit one of our patients that is having issues, and she can't come to us because her legs are too swollen. She's eighty-five and lives with her daughter not far from here," she started, testing for my response.

"Wait. I'll come with you. Can we be back in an hour for our next patient?"

She smiled. "Sure, I know where she lives. I've done this before." I drove, and we talked about the patient and how I admired her for doing this. The visit was documented in the past as a nurse visit – no charge.

"Miss Ellie. This is Doctor Adams, our new doctor," she said as an introduction. Miss Ellie was seated in a recliner with a bible in her lap. The TV was on, and she was wearing a thin pink bathrobe. The recliner elevated her legs. They were so swollen fluid was leaking from the stretched skin to a towel under her legs. Heart failure was the most common cause of this.

"Oh, Doctor Adams, Debbie, your nurse, has told me all about you. She is such a blessing," she said quickly. Her eyes were bright and gleaming, accented by a smile that would melt any heart.

We took her blood pressure and temperature, reviewed her medications, and made a medication change. I called in the change to her pharmacy on my cell phone. She agreed that her daughter would bring her to the clinic in a week for a recheck and lab tests.

As we hugged her goodbye, she pulled a twenty-dollar bill from the bible in her lap and tried to hand it to me. "You're a saint, Doctor. Please take this," she pleaded.

"Miss Ellie, no. We will send a bill to Medicare for a home visit, and they'll pay us. Keep your money, please. And we both enjoyed the visit, so perhaps we can do this again," I said frankly. Hugs and handshakes followed, and we made it back to the clinic on time.

"I understand you went to see Miss Ellie yesterday," said the third patient in a row the following morning.

"I did. But wait; I'm confused. How is it that you and the last two patients this morning know that my nurse and I made a house call yesterday?"

"Doc. Everyone in this town knows you saw Miss Ellie yesterday. After you left her house, she called every Baptist church in town and put you on their prayer lists. You are famous in our Baptist community now," he finished with a big grin. I was a bit stunned. God works in mysterious ways.

That same week, a seventy-three-year-old, white-haired gentleman came to our clinic with his wife. He was a new patient coming in for a physical. I saw him walking into the room and noticed his walk was abnormal. He was flopping his feet and taking short steps. This was classic in conditions like Parkinson's Disease or other neurologic disorders. He was alert and well dressed, and his dark green eyes were bright and watching me closely.

"I just don't feel right, Doctor," he stated. His wife was standing close to him and nodding her head.

"Mr. Nolan let's see what we can find. I'll start at the top and work my way to the bottom. Follow my finger with your eyes," I began and examined everything, but skipped the rectal exam, as he assured me everything was working fine there. He did not have the typical hand tremors seen in Parkinson's Disease. He seemed fine other than his strange gait.

"I don't see anything obvious to worry about here," I reassured. "I'm going to do a full set of standard lab tests now and will add a few extra tests looking for cancer or inflammation. We will also look at your thyroid function. If something is wrong, we'll find it," I concluded.

We shook hands, and I asked them to set up an appointment for the next week so we could go over the labs together and take another look. Something was abnormal. It was Friday afternoon.

I spent that weekend at home with my family. Sunday evening found me thinking about my full schedule on Monday. Perhaps I could make the day better if I reviewed Friday's labs now. That would save time tomorrow, so I logged onto our electronic medical record (EMR) system from home. There were lots of labs to evaluate.

This was taking time on a Sunday evening, and I was trying to finish soon. I rarely check labs on weekends.

In each case, after reviewing a set of normal labs, I would mark them as 'reviewed' and send a pre-written standard note to the patient. If the patient was not enrolled in our EMR system, I would send the same note to the nurse to call the patient with the information.

I came to Mr. Nolan's labs. They were all normal. As I got ready to push 'send' to my nurse, I was hit with a bothersome thought.

Why are they all normal? There was clearly something wrong with his walk, and both he and his wife were concerned. His visit was not just to establish care with a new doctor. They believed something bad was going on.

I did something else I rarely do on the weekend. I picked up the phone and called him.

"Mr. Nolan, this is Doctor Adams. I was reviewing your labs and wanted to call and see how you were doing." I was fishing for more information.

"Doctor, I'm glad you called. I am much worse."

He went on to describe his worsening symptoms. They had been getting worse all weekend, and he could barely walk. His vision was getting worse, and he had a headache that would not go away.

"Sir give the phone to your wife, right now, please," I said decisively.

She came on the phone.

"Mrs. Nolan, I need you to call an ambulance and get your husband to the hospital now," I stated.

"Sir, we have an appointment with you at your clinic tomorrow. He'll be fine until then, I think," she interrupted.

"Ma'am, I think your husband is bleeding inside his head. He may need help that might include surgery tonight. If you don't call right now, I will. He needs to go to the emergency room immediately," I stated as directly as I could. She understood.

"Alright, I'll call as soon as we hang up. Thank you, Doctor Adams." We hung up, and I leaned back and took a deep breath. Bleeding in his head would explain the normal labs, but abnormal and now worsening symptoms. *Thank you, Lord.*

I checked the EMR Monday morning and saw that he had gone to surgery directly from the emergency room. They had done a head CT scan, which showed the intracranial bleeding I had suspected.

One week later, they returned together. His head was half-shaved, and he had an incision that stretched from his forehead to the back of his head. There were metal staples every half of an inch along the left side of his scalp. I admired the surgeon's handiwork.

His wife started. "Doctor Adams, the surgeon that operated on him Sunday night, told us to tell you that the doctor who sent him in that night had saved his life. He said he would not have lived through the night. They removed a baseball-sized blood clot from his head. We can't thank you enough," she reported, amazed.

"Mr. Nolan, I need to tell you that the *Doctor* who saved your life on Sunday was not me. God had a role in our lives that night. I'm still wondering why I did what I did that evening. I don't usually review labs on Sundays or call patients when the labs are all normal. I had an intuition, or I heard a voice, so I believe your *Doctor* was in heaven that night. He directed my thoughts and actions."

They nodded in understanding. "God needs help on earth, you know. You're a saint in our book," smiled the wife. I blushed, remembering God's presence in my life and all the area churches that kept me on their prayer lists. Then a thought hit me.

"Sir, what do you do for a living?"

"I'm a retired minister," he smiled. We have been close ever since.

I asked his blessing at each future visit, which he was always happy to give. God has always been present in my efforts to help others. I touch each patient with warm hands empowered to heal by the prayers and blessings of others.

Chapter 60 - Hypertension – The Mystery

"What's my blood pressure supposed to be?" she began.

"That isn't a simple question to answer. Your age is sixty-two, so that puts you in a different category than your children. Your recommended blood pressure goal is supposed to be higher due to the changes that occur with aging. You and I both have timeworn arteries. They're stiffer, and our organs need the blood and nutrients that must travel along our network of vessels. As a result, our brain, the control center, helps us with higher blood pressures," I begin when talking to my more mature patients.

"I can make your blood pressure be anything I want. We have lots of drugs for that," I continue.

"My goal is to use the fewest medications. This limits side effects and lowers the cost to you. And you need to know that when and how you check your blood pressure is significant. That's why we wait to check your pressure until the last part of checking you in. White coat hypertension is a term for high blood pressure seen because you walked into this office."

I get a tentative nod.

"The best time to check is mid-morning or mid-afternoon, but only after you have been sitting quietly for five minutes. Activity, digesting food, and even reading a book can make your blood pressure rise. Plus, it's important to remember that blood pressure will go up and down all day and night to adjust to your body's needs. So, by definition, we only care to measure blood pressure after five minutes at rest, always sitting, and with your arm resting at heart level."

"But Doc, my blood pressure has been as high as 170 over 100 at times. Isn't that dangerous?" she asks.

I smile and take a deep breath. I have had this same conversation thousands of times. For me it is rehearsed, but accurate.

"No, it isn't dangerous. It's what you're supposed to have if you're active. When we put you on a treadmill and take you for a walk during a cardiac treadmill test, we also monitor your blood pressure. 170/100 is quite normal at that time. It will be lower when you sleep, since your organs don't need extra help then," I explain.

I am watching the clock. It takes a chunk out of a fifteen-minute appointment to explain adequately, but if I don't take the time, the question will keep coming back. When I take the time, it pays dividends. The patients spend less money on drugs they don't need, and they have fewer medication-related issues.

"But my ankles are swelling almost every day. Shouldn't I be on a water pill? My sister takes one."

Here we go again.

"You have worn-out ancient veins," I continue smiling. "Puffy legs are common as we age, due to good ol' gravity having its way with us. The veins leak a bit as the pressure of gravity works on us. This is especially true if we're standing and not walking. Teachers on their feet all day have this puffy ankle problem, but it's not dangerous.

"You ladies want skinny ankles to look good in girl shoes, I understand. But please don't look for drugs to make this happen. I hate girl shoes, by the way. Men designed them to make my doctor-life harder," I grin. "The healthiest way to have skinny ankles is to go for a walk. Your muscles contract with each step and that pushes fluid back into circulation. The lymphatic system does it for you," I add, watching for understanding.

If I see a spark of interest, I continue by rechecking the blood pressure. It is always lower than when the nurse checked it.

"Trust me, please. I don't want you to worry about temporary blips in your blood pressure. You're at the goal we need for good health, and we can avoid the more dangerous problem of low blood pressure," I try to conclude.

"Low blood pressure causes falling down. That leads to broken hips and shoulders, inactivity, pneumonia, and death. As a matter of fact, the leading cause of death in your age group isn't caused by high blood pressure. It's caused by falling."

I listen to her heart and lungs, do a quick exam of ears, throat, eyes, and abdomen and continue my lecture.

"Let me refill your current medicine for you now. Try checking your blood pressure between meals and send me a note if it's too high. And don't smoke a cigarette before you check. Nicotine makes your blood pressure go up like it did today. I can smell the cigarette you had before walking in here."

She nodded.

Chapter 61 – Diabetes – The Epidemic

"Really, Doc, I'm doing everything your dietician told me to do. I don't understand why I'm still gaining weight, and my sugars are worse," she began again. We had the same conversation multiple times. Every three months, she returned and blamed her thyroid, or the medicines, or her horrible job for making her sugars and weight go up.

"Did you drink any sweet tea or soda this month?" She knew this question was coming. I liked her. She came from a large, educated, southern family, and was always polite and attentive. Today she wore an attractive patterned cotton dress to her ankles, and she watched me with alert, dark brown eyes. Her dress was XXXXL.

"Only once, at a work lunch," she lied. "I had some sweet tea. You know, I grew up drinking sweet tea. That was in my bottle as a child. Momma called it juice. I still love it and make my own for the family."

"You cannot have one sip of sweet tea. Ever," I repeated. "It's what causes your diabetes, and it's trying to kill you now. I know you don't like to hear that, but if you don't help, there isn't enough medicine in the world that will control your sugars. Do you know that the fast-food restaurants up north don't even serve sweet tea? The southern tradition, with this horrible drink, requires that the restaurants boil the tea, so more sugar will dissolve in it. They supersaturate the tea. Your brain gets a sugar rush, and you get fat."

"What am I supposed to drink? Water?" she asks.

"Most anything is better -- except for Mountain Dew. That's the other cause of diabetes in this town," I noted.

"I know. You told me that before, but honestly, I'm not sure I can live a life without sweet tea," she concludes with a pleading look.

I did not see much diabetes in my military patients or families. That population needed to be fit, and they were. Now this disease was taking over the biscuit-loving South.

"I drive to work each morning at 7 AM and pass Chick-Fil-A and Krispy Kreme Donuts in the same block as our clinic. There's a line around both buildings with patients getting their ninety-nine-cent extra-large sweet tea and biscuits or a dozen hot donuts. It makes me smile because I know that I will never run out of patients," I ended in mock disgust.

"Sure, I get it. But, I have to tell you that in our family, for as long as I can remember, we have never gone out to a restaurant that did not have the word 'buffet' in it," she added as if that explanation would relieve her of responsibility.

"OK, I hear you. But please hear me. You are 425 pounds today, and that is up another five pounds from your last visit. You're on huge doses of medicine and insulin, and your sugars are still uncontrolled."

She nodded again with understanding, but no remorse.

"We're going to start seeing bad things happen soon. You will lose your vision, your feet are going to go numb, your heart is working overtime already, and strokes are more likely. We are going to start amputating toes first, and then your feet, if we can't get you to help more," I pleaded.

"I'll try Doc. Really, I will," she always said. We both know she does not mean it.

One year later, she came in to see me. She had had two toes amputated because of a common diabetic condition called dry gangrene. Her toes had lost circulation, and they turned hard and dark black. They had lost feeling long ago, and now they were dead.

"OK, I'm ready to do something now. Can I have gastric bypass surgery?" she questioned.

"Yes, you can, but that means you couldn't go to a buffet restaurant ever again. As a matter of fact, you wouldn't be able to eat much at all. Can you deal with a life like that? Can you even imagine what you would do with your family that wants to spend much of their waking hours eating?" I asked, with concern in my voice.

"I have to do it now. It's time," she whispered.

Surgery worked. She lost 220 pounds in the next two years, her sugars improved, we got her off insulin, and she smiled more often. It was fun to see her get better.

Two years later, she was back, after a six-month absence, and we noted that she had gained thirty pounds.

"What's going on? Why did you miss your last appointment?" I wondered out loud.

"I got tired of not eating. It sucked. I'm taking the medicines, but I seriously missed my ice cream and desserts. I knew that my sugar would be worse, but dang Doc, I don't want to live like this."

I nodded in understanding, reminded her that I was always there for her, reviewed the treatment plan, and requested she let me keep helping. She agreed to try again.

The next day a petite Southern woman presented for evaluation of her symptoms of chronic thirst, weight loss, and urinating all the time - day and night. To my surprise, she was not overweight since she probably had diabetes with a classic presentation.

"I have your Hemoglobin A1C results from the finger-stick lab the nurse did," I began. I had her attention. "It shows that you have uncontrolled diabetes and is almost high enough to justify admitting you to the hospital to get it under control." I paused, and she nodded, looking confused.

"Do you drink sweet tea?" I ventured as a start to the conversation I was having routinely.

"Oh, yes! It's my favorite food. I have it three meals a day and at work," she responded with enthusiasm.

"Well, frankly, you can't ever drink sweet tea again," I began to get her attention. It worked.

The loud wailing emanating from the room caused my nurse to run in. "What did you do to her?" she demanded with concern.

"Nothing!" I replied defensively. "I just told her she couldn't drink sweet tea anymore." The loud crying continued. "I'm going to step out for a minute and let you talk to her about a diabetic diet now," I mumbled. Exiting quickly, I paused in the hallway to find the staff all looking at me. I had no idea then that this drink was so ingrained in the Southern diet that it literally defined food choices daily.

Children can get Type 2 diabetes from too much sugar also, but the more common form is Type 1 diabetes that results from a viral infection leading to the inability of the pancreas to make insulin. These children get extremely sick with chronic thirst, hunger, and frequent urination. They are usually quite thin and commonly diagnosed from two to fourteen years old. The only treatment is supplemental insulin. In the emergency room one evening a dad brought his extremely thin six-year old daughter in for weight loss, thirst and urinating all the time. Her glucose level came back at 600 which is critically high. "Sir, the nurse tells me you do not have medical insurance," I began. "Yes but do whatever you need to do. I am so sorry I waited to bring her in," he pleaded.

"I am going to admit her to our pediatric ICU and we will get her better. But I am not going to write 'diabetes' on her chart today so you can avoid pre-existing illness issues with insurance. She will need expensive insulin for the rest of her life. There is no cure for this. So, if you can get insurance today, I would strongly recommend doing so." He nodded in understanding, but I never discovered if he got it.

Chapter 62 – Mentor – Three Years After Residency

"I don't understand why my patient will not stop drinking Pepsi. It's killing her. She kind of freaked out when I asked her to lose weight by following a better diet. How am I supposed to help her? She's grossly obese, and won't stop eating," Doctor Shea noted with frustration and anger in her voice.

Doctor Shea was a brilliant and caring doctor. Her patients loved her and brought her gifts, and she treated them as part of her family. She remembered what her teachers had taught her and used online expert resources to verify what she knew. Her advice was always reasonable and 'by the book.'

I knew how she felt. It was a common frustration when a patient made bad or even dangerous choices. I considered my response, which I had given to other younger doctors before.

"Liz, your patients have a right to make bad life choices. You need to understand and accept that. It's unproductive for you to take it personally. What's going to happen is that one day your patient will come to realize you care. It might take a few visits, or it might take a few years. In the meantime, you keep educating, explaining the benefits, and letting them know you're giving advice to help them."

I paused to let that sink in. "Your patients will smoke and die too young. They know they'll die young. Others will remain out-of-control diabetics, until they go partially blind, or start losing toes to amputation. It won't be your fault," I continued.

"I start every day hoping another patient will show up and tell me they had an 'ah-ha' moment. They realize that the advice we're giving them is useful. They'll try it, and it'll work. It will happen when they're ready. A life event will cause them to think about what you say and what they want. Unexpectedly, they'll come in with better blood pressure, weight loss, and a smile. They'll thank you for your advice. That's when we should try to reinforce their good choices. We just gave them the necessary information," I finished.

The next week Liz came to ask me about a patient I had advised not to take a statin medicine for her cholesterol. She reminded me that 'the book' says she must take it.

"Liz, in about another year or so, you will realize that 'the book' is a guideline. What our teachers taught us were guidelines. Residency was like three years drinking from a firehose, exposing us to the basic principles of medicine. You're now in the early years following residency. This is the time you become a real doctor. You're learning that the guidelines don't apply to everyone. You're learning from your patients. It will continue for the rest of your life, and they'll teach you what works. They'll show you how to be the best healthcare advocate you can be," I lectured kindly.

"No one told me this when I started practicing on my own. I called one of my residency teachers one day and told him I was interested and confused that I was not practicing the way he had taught me," I continued.

"You have been on your own now for over three years," he reminded me. "That's when doctors have enough patient experience to start practicing patient-based care. From this point on, your patients become your teachers. You will learn from them what works best. Welcome to the club," he concluded.

She heard what I said, nodded her head, and walked away with a contemplative look on her face. One year later, she stopped me in the hallway.

"Bob, you were right. I'm not using 'the book' now. I'm doing what's right for my patients, and they're getting better care." She was as pleased as I had been when I had made the same discovery years before.

The practice of good medicine is an art, and it begins by listening to our patients. They will tell us what we need to know to help them.

Chapter 63 - DSAP the First Time

"It looks like we're making progress. We can freeze off a few more today," I stated cheerfully.

"Yes, but I wonder if these will come back again. I've had these things for most of my life," she observed.

That made me wonder. I was in a hurry and making progress using liquid nitrogen to freeze the skin lesions that covered both arms. There were a few more on her legs too. They looked and felt like sun-damaged skin lesions called actinic keratosis. The odd thing was she was too young to have sun-damaged skin, and there were too many of them.

"You know, I don't know the answer to your question because truthfully, I don't understand what these skin things actually are or what's causing them. I would like to know why they're here. Would you mind if I did a biopsy and sent it off to a pathologist to analyze? Maybe we can find out what's causing this."

"Sure," she replied gratefully.

We moved to the procedure room, and I injected her with numbing medicine and used a five-millimeter skin punch device to sample the edge of the most prominent lesion. I cauterized the hole to stop the small amount of bleeding and placed a Band-Aid over the biopsy site.

The result arrived two days later. It read in part, "consider Disseminated Superficial Actinic Keratosis."

What?

That took me to my dermatology book.

"I think I may know what those spots on your arm are," I began after dialing her number.

"What?" she asked.

"Let me ask you something first. Does anyone in your family have the same skin spots?"

"Yes, my mother does. But she doesn't know what causes them either."

"In that case, you will want to write this down. You and your mother have an inherited condition known as DSAP. I'll spell it for you, and, honestly, you are the first person I have ever met with this condition. The good news is it's not harmful, and we can keep freezing spots to help with the cosmetics," I stated proudly.

The next month another female patient of mine came in for her routine blood pressure check, and I noticed her arms. She had the same kind of skin spots.

"Does anyone in your family have those dry skin spots like you have on your arms?"

"Yes, my mom and sister both have them. They don't bother me."

"Do you know why you have them, or what they're called?" I asked.

"No. We just think we inherited dry skin."

I went on to explain that she did have an inherited condition, and it was called DSAP. I offered to treat it, but she refused.

"Honestly, they don't bother me. I use moisturizing creams. But I'll tell my sister and mother that it has a name if you will write that down for me."

A few months later, a woman came in for her physical, and I noticed that her legs were covered with similar lesions. She also had DSAP. Now that I knew what it was, I started to notice it on patients that I had seen before.

If you don't know what you don't know, it is challenging to discover what you need to know. Once you see something new, you will almost always recognize it again. Then you know what you did not know.

"I don't know what's wrong with you. But there's nothing new in medicine. Someone has already had whatever is causing your symptoms. Give me time, and we will figure this out," I start when faced with something new or confusing.

"Let me do lab tests today, and then come back in a week or two, so we can review them, and I can do another exam. We may need to do an ultrasound if the labs don't help."

"I hate not knowing *why* something is happening, so work with me, please, and we'll figure it out. Somewhere there's a book with your symptoms in it. We need more clues to find that book. And after your next visit, if I can't figure it out, we can ask a specialist to take a look also," I say to reassure my patient and give her hope.

This always leads to a diagnosis. Sometimes it just takes time.

Chapter 64 - Did You Save a Life Today?

"Honey, I'm home," is my standard greeting walking in the door.

"Did you save a life today?" is a common follow-up question.

"Let me think. Well, yes, I did."

"A forty-year-old male auto-worker named David Hempstead came in this morning for his new-patient physical. He smoked two packs a day and was on no medications. His wife had sent him in for his physical, and he thought he was fine. His blood pressure was elevated a bit at 155/85, but in taking his history, he told me that he had experienced a few events of chest pain in the recent past. That was one reason his wife sent him," I noted, starting the story.

"His physical exam was normal, and I was going to send him for labs and a follow-up, but wives are always worth paying attention to, *as you know Dear*, so I ordered an EKG. The results surprised me since he was only forty years old," I continued.

"I was amazed when I looked at it, and then I asked him, when did you have your heart attack? And he just said, *What?*"

"According to his EKG, he had already had at least one heart attack, as he had Q-waves in all the leads, and that says *heart attack*. So I told him I thought that his past chest pains had been an actual heart attack. The good news was that he was alive to talk about it, so I made a phone call to my favorite cardiologist, and he was able to see him today. They admitted him, and he had a heart catheterization this afternoon. They scheduled him for a triple bypass heart surgery tomorrow. One life saved," I finished proudly.

David did well after his surgery and stopped smoking immediately. He was one of the youngest open-heart surgery patients I ever had.

Another day began with one of my more difficult diabetics. She was a smoker, and I had reminded her of the risks many times. Those risks included multiple cancers.

As I listened to her heart, with my stethoscope on her chest, I noticed a small black area of skin on her left breast.

"How long has that been there?" I asked, pointing to the irregular black area of skin. It was small, but suspicious for the worst kind of skin cancer.

"I don't know," she answered, looking down. "I don't remember seeing it before."

I had a full schedule that day with no open appointment slots. I knew the rest of the week was the same. The lesion needed to be biopsied. A referral to a dermatologist would take weeks.

"OK. We're moving you to the procedure room now," I explained. "This could be a malignant melanoma. Skin cancers are more common in smokers," I reminded her.

"It might be the bad kind of skin cancer, so we'll remove it now. It may take a little time to get set up, but we're going to do it today," I finished. She nodded.

The biopsy came back the next day. It confirmed, *malignant melanoma in situ, margins clear*. By removing it completely, she was cured. Life saved. She eventually quit smoking -- a life saved twice.

Experiences like these are remarkably common. You don't need to be in an emergency room to save a life. Heart attacks, respiratory failure, infections, lacerations, strokes, seizures, and many other life-threatening presentations come to family medicine offices daily.

Chapter 65 – Oxycodone and Heroin

"Doc, I think it's time to stop using heroin," he stated evenly and logically.

This caught me by surprise. The well-dressed forty-two-year-old gentleman sat primly in my exam room and spoke matter-of-factly.

"Oh," I stammered. "How often are you using heroin, sir?"

"Every day, for some time now," he responded.

Unsure of where to take the conversation, I continued. "That must be expensive. How much are you spending on heroin?"

"About $100,000 a year. That is one reason it's time to stop," he continued smiling.

"Dang. How do you afford that?" I continued fascinated.

"I have a good income. I own a paving company," was his quiet reply.

The fifteen-minute office visit ended without a plan. This drug typically owned a person, body and soul.

I suggested the six-week inpatient rehabilitation facility option and ordered basic laboratory tests to ensure he was healthy enough to go through withdrawal intervention, but I never saw him again. I believe he was there that day to see if anyone had come up with a newer more natural way. He discovered there was no easy option.

That same month, I received a phone call from a close friend.

"Bob, you gotta help me. I'm going to California to bring my son back. He's living in a field in a pup tent, addicted to heroin. He works just enough in restaurants to get money for his drugs. He's covered head-to-toe with sores. The police tell me they can't help because drug use in California isn't considered a crime anymore. I plan to put him on a plane and bring him home here to Wisconsin, where he'll have family and church support."

"Tom, you will have a hard time with this. Is he willing to come home?" I asked.

"I'm not sure, but he knows I'm coming. What do I do if he goes through withdrawal on the plane?" he stammered.

"His symptoms will begin eight hours after his last dose. That's when he'll be in trouble, and you'll have a hard time managing his anxiety, sweating, diarrhea, and inability to sleep. He'll be climbing the walls for about 48 hours. Methadone treatment is an option if you can get him to a clinic there. But, Tom, I gotta warn you that you're likely to fail unless he wants your help," I concluded.

Two weeks later, I learned that his son was off the drug, living at home, and starting to look for a job. I was thrilled and amazed.

Three months after that, Tom called me in tears. He said his son had saved enough money for a plane ticket and had gone back to California. He missed his heroin too much.

Oxycodone, Fentanyl, Xanax, and more are available on the street and are killer drugs doctors eventually must deal with. Family physicians are frequently the first persons a patient comes to for a refill of their narcotic pain or anxiety medicine. Often, the drug was started by a well-meaning orthopedic surgeon, general surgeon, or hospitalist. They would do their jobs and send patients home with ten days of oxycodone or Xanax and a note to follow-up with their primary care physician.

Ten days is plenty of time to become dependent.

"Doc, seriously, my knee is killing me. I can't sleep and just walking hurts. Nothing else helps. I've tried it all. I need a refill, please. It stops the pain," they plead.

The words are almost always the same. It is routinely a battle -- often an unpleasant one -- to get them to accept alternatives for pain or anxiety management.

"I was cleaning my gutters and fell off the ladder. My back is killing me," he started.

"Show me where it hurts," I probed.

He pointed to his low back. I lifted his shirt and saw no bruise or abrasion.

"Let me check something on my computer," I paused, and then entered his name in the state-mandated narcotic prescription tracking database.

"Sir, I see you have received narcotic medication from three different doctors in the last two months. I'm sorry to tell you that you won't be getting any here today. But let me make a suggestion, please. We have been successful in the past, helping patients stop using these costly and addictive medicines. If you want help today or in the future, all you need to do is ask. We can help," I concluded with passion.

He nodded and left. I never saw him again.

That same month a visitor came in and asked to see me. The front desk knew him well. He and his wife had been our patients for years. He had completed six months of inpatient and supervised heroin addiction treatment, and he wanted to let us know.

"Doctor Adams. You remember Darrell Shifflett and his wife, don't you?" began our receptionist.

"He's at the front window and wants to see you. He's back from rehab and looks good," she finished smiling.

"Of course. I'll be right there," I answered.

I opened the door and asked him to step into the more private clinic area.

"Darrell, how are you?"

"Doc, I'm a lot better. I have my life back. It has been a pretty horrible experience. My church and family have been behind me all the way, and I'm clean. I go to Narcotics Anonymous almost daily now, and I have custody of the kids," he shared.

"Custody? Does that mean you're separated? What happened?" I whispered.

"She couldn't do it, Doc. She tried. It was awful to watch her go through withdrawal for days. She screamed and shook and went almost insane. We all tried to help, and after three days in the house, she appeared like she might be OK. But she went back to heroin. She's lost and living with other addicts now. I got the house out of foreclosure with help from dad, and the kids and I are OK. I wanted you all to know that I made it," he finished softly and proudly.

They had tried heroin one time together. That was all it took to get hooked. He beat the odds, with help from family, church, and prolonged professional inpatient services. His wife did not.

It is a joyful event each time he comes back to see us.

Chapter 66 - Led Ford Story

Led had been my fishing buddy for six years when he finally told me about his military experiences in Vietnam. He had grown up very poor in Florida, where he fished and hunted with a slingshot for food.

We had met when he answered my ad in the Sporting Goods section of the local paper, looking for places to fish. My first duty station after completing the three-year residency training was in Fayetteville, NC. There were lakes and rivers all around, but where to go was a mystery.

"Hey, are you the guy that put an ad in the paper about fishing?" Led began with his thick Southern accent.

"Yes, I am."

"Well, that is the funniest ad I have ever read. I fish every day. When do you want to go?" he asked seriously.

"How about this Saturday," I proposed.

"Great, I'll pick you up at 6 AM," he chuckled. And for the next six years, we fished often. I would tell him about my Army life as a doctor, my past Navy life, and even a bit about working with DELTA Force. All he said was that he had done a tour in Vietnam, and the Veterans Administration had treated him rudely when he got out. He never went back to them.

Led was a powerful man with a working man's hands that barely knew their own strength. He could shoot a gun and a bow and arrow with uncanny accuracy. He carved intricate models of birds in flight from scrap wood. His innate ability to see a better way led to inventions that made things work more efficiently. He was the first in his family to graduate high school and was drafted when the war came. In boot camp, he gained weight and grew two inches. Eating three meals a day was a new experience.

He returned from war and married the woman of his dreams. They adopted children that have blessed them with grandchildren. Their extended family remains close and interdependent. Led and his wife represent what makes America special: love and devotion to family and community.

He also had medical issues, including horrible asthma and respiratory sensitivity to smoke and fumes. He rarely slept. He would work or fish at night until he got tired enough to collapse into bed and sleep. He had been sleeping two hours every two nights for the last thirty-five years. His wife and grandchildren knew not to wake him as he would often awaken confused and violent.

"Doc, you're in the Army. Can you tell me what this is, please?" he asked one late afternoon after our fishing trip. We were in his neat home. They adorned the walls with mounted catfish, bass, and crappie that were award-winning sizes. He held out a piece of paper.

I read the words with amazement.

"Led, this is your Bronze Star Medal citation from Vietnam. It says you were a machine gunner, and one of the few survivors of your unit, when a large enemy force overran it," I stated with confusion in my voice.

"Why are you showing me this?" I whispered.

"Doc, seriously, I don't think that is me. I don't remember anything like that at all," he added, confused.

Oh, no! I thought. Suddenly, his symptoms made sense. He had severe PTSD, and I had missed that all these years. *No wonder he would not talk to me about his military past.*

"Led, this is you, and awful stuff happened to you according to this. You have blocked it out of your memory. But it explains to me why you've been having trouble sleeping, and many of the other symptoms I've been treating. If you let me, I would like to start you on a medicine that can help you sleep and feel better," I ventured cautiously.

We had been friends long enough now that he trusted me, so I started him on an antidepressant once a day and waited to see if it would help.

He called ten days later.

"Doc, my wife, Mary, told me to call you. I slept six hours last night. I don't ever remember doing that. You're a miracle worker, and I have energy again. Please promise me you will keep giving me this medicine," he finished in a frantic voice.

Led continued to get better. Thirty-five years of PTSD had affected him in so many ways. He could not be in elevators or crowds. He remembered being warned in Vietnam that a group of three or more men standing together became a target. His memory was poor, and he had horrible anxiety issues.

He was brilliant, an inventor with admirable skills, and at work, he fixed things. As a tire line-worker, his mechanical improvements to his machines made him the top producer by a large margin. He saw mechanical things and knew how to make them work better. They offered him promotions, which he always turned down. His hands were muscular and substantial, yet he carved me a tiny intricate bird in flight from dark wood. I admire and treasure it in wonder that his hands could create such art.

He had felt safe as a loner and would often go fishing at night because he could not sleep more than two hours at a time.

"Led, it's time to go back to the Veterans Administration," I started. He recoiled.

"Look, you're not a rich man, and you've got a wife, kids, and grandkids to help. The VA owes you long-overdue help, and they can provide that for free. Also, and this is important, you're eligible for compensation for your condition. They pay disability benefits to you monthly, and it's free of taxes. It could be significant," I concluded.

"What do I need to do?" he asked reluctantly.

"You need to fill out a form. I have printed it out for you. All you have to do is answer the questions about the unit they assigned you to and make a brief statement about what happened the day they attacked your unit.

He agreed, and I gave him the three-page form to complete.

Two weeks later, I called to ask if he was done with the form.

"I can't do it. I've tried. I just can't think about that time and make the words come. I'm sorry, Doc," he whispered.

"OK, Led, no problem. Let's do it together. I have a copy of the form here. All you need to do is tell me the story of what happened, and I'll fill in the form for you. We only need one traumatic event to document a place and time. Why don't you start with your job as a machine gunner? Tell me about what happened that day."

By the time I stopped him, he was sobbing uncontrollably, and tears welled up in my eyes too. I was stunned. He had endured combat at its worst, and I had seven different horrible events documented. Any one of them would qualify him for the diagnosis of PTSD.

I took him the forms to review and sign, and we mailed them to the local Veterans Administration.

Led is now one hundred percent disabled and receiving VA compensation. He worked hard and retired from his tire job after forty years on the line. He enrolled in a PTSD counseling group, which he attends faithfully, and he is doing well on medication. I moved away, but we still fish together and trade Christmas presents.

I kick myself for taking six years to make his diagnosis.

Chapter 67 - Kallmann Syndrome

"Bob, I'm sending you a patient next week that I don't know what to do with. She came in today, asking for help to get pregnant," stated the nurse practitioner. We worked in the same clinic, and I was her supervising physician. She was recently out of school and enjoying the learning experiences of a busy full-service clinic. Women preferred to see her despite her relative inexperience because she listened.

"The issue that concerns me is that she's twenty-two years old and has never had a period," she concluded.

"OK, you got my attention with that one. What did you do?"

"I ordered all the hormone labs and told her to come back to see you to review labs and do the pap smear and physical exam. She seemed happy with that plan," she finished hopefully.

"Good job. I'll let you know what I find. It should be interesting," I smiled.

The next week, the patient presented for her physical. My nurse had her undress in the exam room and cover herself with a paper sheet. I entered the room with my nurse to introduce myself but had not seen her chart yet.

"Hello, Mrs. Tanner, I'm Doctor Adams, and we're going to start with the exam and pap smear today. After that, we can discuss the pregnancy issue. Is that OK?"

"Yes, Doctor," she said from the exam table, lying flat, head on a pillow. She had bright blond hair, a perfect complexion, and appeared thin, but well.

"I'm going to do a quick breast exam to start," I stated as I rolled the blue paper sheet down from her right shoulder to reveal the breast.

It surprised me to see a tiny breast with a small, almost male nipple. "You have small breasts," I commented casually, as I went through the standard motions of a breast exam. She nodded, and my nurse watched me with a watchful gaze. I thought about her absence of a period and wondered to myself what I might find at the other end. I remembered she was married and reported having intercourse. *There must be a vagina there.*

"We're going to do the pap smear next," I stated, moving to the small metal stool placed at the foot of the table. I pulled out the retractable foot stirrups and asked her to scoot down the table and put her feet in the stirrups. She complied watchfully and expertly.

The nurse handed me a small size speculum used to look inside the vagina. It was coated lightly with a clear lubricant.

"This is going to feel chilly. I'm putting extra lubrication here," I commented as I wiped K-Y Jelly on the vaginal area and placed my index finger inside the vaginal opening and gently pushed downward.

"I want you to relax this muscle, please. I'm going to insert a small-size lubricated speculum now," I explained.

The speculum was plastic and had its own light source. It allowed me a good view of the vaginal wall and the cervix. The cervix is the only visible part of the uterus, and it was unusually small. I was surprised again.

"You have a very small cervix," I observed, while I brushed the cervix with the small brush used for pap smears.

"Yes. I have infantile adnexa," she responded knowingly. She caught me by surprise once more.

"We're done with the pap. I'm going to step out while my nurse helps you clean up and get dressed. Then, I'll be back to go over your labs with you."

When I came back in, she was sitting primly in the clinic chair. She was young, healthy, and watchful.

"Let's look at these labs together," I started as I flipped open her brown paper, hand-written chart. Her labs had been printed and added into the lab section. She leaned forward.

"Now, this is interesting. All your basic labs like blood count and electrolytes are normal, but the follicle-stimulating hormone (FSH) and luteinizing hormone (LH) are both quite low. I have never seen this before," I stated. "I need a minute to look it up."

I grabbed my reference book for interpreting laboratory values and flipped to the pages for LH and FSH. There was a long list of diagnoses that would be considered if these lab values were high or low. Her LH and FSH values were 'zero.' This is unimaginable in a patient with ovaries, which I was pretty sure she had.

At the bottom of the page, I noticed a postscript. "If the patient has very low, or zero, LH and FSH, consider Kallmann Syndrome. These patients typically cannot smell."

I turned toward my patient with new interest and asked, "Ma'am, can you smell?"

"Oh no, sir. I have anosmia." I was astonished she knew the medical word and its meaning. I remembered her use of *infantile adnexa* and realized past doctors must have identified these findings without addressing their cause.

I had made the diagnosis of Kallmann Syndrome and told her so.

I had no idea what we would do now, but I would find out and get back with her. She was accepting and left.

After my last patient that morning, I researched more about Kallmann Syndrome and realized I would need help from a specialist. I called my favorite gynecologist and asked who I should talk to. She had never heard of this before either but suggested I contact a gynecologic endocrinologist. I was unaware such a specialist existed. She said to call Duke Hospital, not far away, in Durham, NC.

After researching the condition, I learned that it was a developmental abnormality. It affected the release of gonadotrophic releasing hormone (GnRH) from the hypothalamus in the brain. The hypothalamus sends chemical orders to the pituitary gland in the brain. The pituitary, in turn, sends luteinizing hormone and follicle-stimulating hormone to the female organs, so they will grow, develop, and function.

The genetic defect that affects the proper growth of the hypothalamic gland also affects the development of the nasal olfactory bulbs that allow for the sense of smell.

"Sir, thank you for taking my call," I began. "I have a patient that I think has Kallmann Syndrome." I proceeded to outline her history and laboratory findings, and before I finished, he interrupted me.

"Holy moly! That is Kallmann Syndrome. That's always a question on my specialty board exam, and I've never seen one. Please let me see her. I can get her in immediately," he begged with excitement.

"Absolutely. I'll send you a formal consult and let her know to expect a call from your office. But help me understand something. Can she get pregnant?"

"Yes, she can. What we do is start her on birth control pills. Remember that the LH and FSH direct the ovaries to produce estrogen and progesterone. Since the ovaries are not getting that signal, they're dormant - asleep and waiting to be turned on. We will introduce the ovarian hormones with birth control pills, and her breasts and uterus will begin to mature."

"Wait," I interrupted. How is she going to get pregnant on birth control pills?"

"That is the amazing part. After her organs mature, we stop the birth control hormones and introduce the drug Clomid to induce ovulation. Then the eggs get released, get fertilized, and implant in a now-adult uterus. Once the uterus responds to implantation - and here comes the cool part - the uterus and ovaries produce enough hormones to maintain the pregnancy," he chuckled, as he finished his lecture.

She came by the office about six months later and wanted to show me her new breasts. I grabbed a nurse chaperone and went into an exam room. She was both pleased and displeased.

As she undid her shirt and bra, to display her now adult-sized breasts and nipples, she said, "I know I need these, but I'm not sure I like them. They hurt, especially around the time of my periods. And I might add, it seems like I had it pretty good, not having periods. They're not my favorite thing either," but she smiled.

I lost track of her after that as she had moved out of state, but I called the GYN endocrine doctor, about a year later, and he confirmed that they had left the area. Then he added proudly that she was pregnant when she left.

Chapter 68 – Oh, By the Way, Doc

The most engaging sentences a patient will say begin with, "Oh, by the way." These words are almost always uttered as I am leaving the room. The patient would have allowed me to run through the medications and refills and abnormal laboratory tests. As I concluded that I had handled all the critical matters of the day, stood up, and moved to the door, the dreaded words would be uttered.

"Oh, by the way, Doc."

"I have a lump in my breast."

"I'm wondering why I can't feel my feet."

"Should I have been having my period for three weeks now?"

"Did your nurse tell you that I've been hearing voices at night?"

"I read that you might be able to inject my knee with steroids to help with my knee pain."

"Did you see my MRI with the pancreatic mass?"

Never ignore these particular words. They often represent the real reason the patient is seeking care. They are always schedule killers.

The proper thing to do is stop, sit back down, and listen.

"Doc, I know you're in a hurry, but my wife wanted me to ask you about a mole on my shoulder," began my last patient of the day. It was 4:55 PM, and we closed at 5 PM.

"Absolutely, sir. I love skin stuff. Let's take a look," I said as I replaced my portable computer onto the desk.

He lifted his shirt and t-shirt to reveal a back covered with brownish waxy lesions. These were benign seborrheic keratoses, which I liked to call *old people barnacles.*

"Where is the spot you're referring to?" I asked.

"I can't see it, but my wife says there's a darker spot on my right shoulder," he added apologetically.

There it was — a black, irregularly shaped, flat lesion hidden among the other blemishes.

"Dang," I muttered.

"What?" he responded.

"I don't like the looks of that dark spot either. It needs a biopsy to make sure it isn't a bad kind of skin cancer," I said with concern.

My thoughts spun. *"It's closing time. A referral to the dermatologist down the street is quick and easy, but she won't get him in soon. He's my last patient today, and I have a pile of notes to finish. My nurse is going to be upset."*

"Alexia, we're moving to the procedure room," I said to my nurse sitting at her desk nearby.

"I need to do a quick skin biopsy. Let the front desk know I'll be running late, and someone needs to stay to check him out. You can take off if you want. I can do it alone," I finished.

"I'll be right there," she responded with a smile.

I knew that was what she would say. I was blessed with a great and caring staff. She was the sunshine in my clinic life.

The shiny stainless tray was already set up for skin biopsies. Alexia flowed brightly into the room after informing the front desk of our plan.

"Lidocaine with epinephrine, 3 cc's?" she asked.

"Yes, please, with a ½ inch 27-gauge needle," I responded gratefully.

"That is already on the tray," she grinned.

"Take off your shirt and t-shirt, please, sir. Alexia has a consent form for you to sign. It confirms that you're not allergic to lidocaine and that the biopsy will hurt a bit, bleed some, and come with a small risk of infection. But, in the years I have been doing these, I have not seen an infection," I stated by rote, as I cleaned the small blackish spot on his shoulder with an alcohol swab.

After witnessing the consent form, Alexia, with newly rubber-gloved hands, moved over and handed me the syringe. She looked at the spot with me and reached for the small formalin-containing sample bottle. She removed the plastic top and placed it on the tray. Then she labeled the bottle with our patient's name and grabbed gauze to dab blood.

"This is the part that is going to sting a bit," I stated. "It will only last a few seconds."

"There. You're numb already," I stated knowingly, as I reached for the flexible biopsy device.

It took ten seconds to shave the entire lesion, plus ½ centimeter of the healthy surrounding skin. I went deep enough to ensure the deep margins would be clear of pigment.

"Done," I announced as Alexia scraped the skin on my blade into the plastic bottle in her hand. "There was no dark pigment that I can see under this piece of skin. That's good. Sometimes when we catch it early, even if it is malignant melanoma, this procedure is a cure," I stated.

"Now, I'm going to use the electrocautery needle to stop this little bit of bleeding. This helps to kill any abnormal cells that might be hanging out around the biopsy area. You will hear a buzzing and smell a burning odor," I mentored by rote. He reeked of cigarette smoke, so I did not believe the new odor would bother him.

Alexia finished by placing a sterile Bacitracin-dabbed dressing on the biopsy site.

"The lab is closed now, so this won't go out until the morning," I declared, holding up the small plastic container with the skin chunk floating in the preservative. "I'll get the results back soon, and I'll call you with the results. If it's the bad kind of skin cancer, which I do suspect, there might be another surgery in your future. If it comes back superficial, *in situ,* we may have saved your life today," I finished smiling.

"Oh, by the way. Please thank your wife for reminding you to ask about this. And, as I said before, please keep trying to stop smoking."

He nodded guiltily, and Alexia escorted him to the front desk. I moved to my office to order the surgical pathology test and finish my notes for the day. It was 5:20 PM, and I felt good about it.

The biopsy results came back to my inbox the next day as *malignant melanoma in situ, margins clear. Wow.* I called the patient with the news, knowing he would be worried.

The next day started with twenty-three patients on my schedule. I was alert and invigorated. Each day brought a new opportunity to help, teach, and learn. *What a great job.*

The second patient of the morning is always a thirty-minute physical. I do not need that long. We get to chat a bit about life and stress. Everyone has life stresses to some degree.

"OK, here is your printed summary. It lists the labs we're doing today. I'll get the results back this afternoon and send you an email with the results. You get another A-plus on your exam, but I reserve the right to change your score once I get your labs back," I add with a smile, and a handshake.

"Sure, Doc. Thanks. Um…. did your nurse tell you there was something else?" he mumbled.

I paused at the door, observed his face now in distress, and closed the door. "What else did you need?" I started with renewed interest. Until now, it was routine.

"I did not want to tell your nurse, but I can't get an erection anymore," he added with concern.

"Is it the medicine or is my testosterone low?" he continued.

This led to a schedule-killing discussion I often have with patients at the end of a regular visit. It was important, and I could help.

The next patient would have to wait a few minutes, and Alexia would knock on the door soon to hurry me along.

Chapter 69 – Mistakes

"He's had a headache for three days, and it isn't going away with Tylenol or Motrin," began the father. He had brought his thirteen-year-old son in to see me because he trusted me. I had been his doctor for many years.

"He plays football at school but hasn't had any bad collisions in practice, and the regular season hasn't started yet. He hasn't had any other symptoms like vomiting or vision changes, but he goes to sleep with a headache and wakes up with one, and I did not let him go to practice yesterday. Thank you so much for accepting him as a new patient."

"I'm honored, sir. Is he on any medications or taking any performance supplements?" I began.

"No, sir."

I did a thorough history and physical exam checking everything I could think of. This was not a typical presentation for a boy his age, but I found nothing at all abnormal.

"Let's get some lab work to check for infection, inflammation, bleeding, thyroid, or other weird and unusual issues," I began in frustration. "I agree with you that something's not exactly feeling right here, and I want to see him back in two weeks. I'll call you tomorrow with the lab results, but I want to see him right away if the headaches get worse or any new symptoms develop. Thank you for bringing him in to me, Jim," I finished as we all walked down the hall to the lab.

"OK, Doc, thanks."

The following week my nurse grabbed me when I came in and told me that the young boy, we had seen the week before, had died. I was stunned. She did not have any other details, so I looked in his hospital records. I knew I would have to call the father soon, but I would wait a day due to the confusion likely going on at his home.

"Doctor Adams, the father of the boy that died yesterday, is on the phone for you," said our front desk staff who peeked her head into my clinic room. I was with a patient, but this had priority, so I excused myself.

"Doc, this is Jim. I guess you heard about my son?" he began.

"Yes, sir. I am so sorry. I looked at his hospital record yesterday and was shocked. I have never ever heard of a brain aneurysm in a child his age."

"I know. That is why I'm calling. I know you're probably beating yourself up over this, and I need you to know that the neurosurgeon told me that he had never seen this in someone so young, either. Please don't blame yourself."

I was bewildered for a moment. "Jim, I don't know what to say. You're calling *me* to see if *I* am OK? I was planning to call you this afternoon to see how you were doing. I just don't believe this happened when all the tests were so normal," I muttered with pain in my voice.

We spoke as friends-in-mourning for a bit more, but Jim never came back to see me as a patient. It would be too hard to revisit his loss and grief.

I worried more in the years that followed about headaches, and I ordered more CT scans than were probably medically indicated.

"I have never had a vasectomy fail yet," I began when counseling my patient. "But one out of 500 vasectomies do fail for various reasons, so your odds are good. I should note, however, that you are my 500th vasectomy." I used this joke routinely when counseling patients prior to this procedure.

An email much later, from the wife of this same patient, had an address that began with 'SixKidsMom@.' She was asking me to schedule another vasectomy for her husband. I had done his vasectomy the previous year when they had only five children. It had obviously failed as she had just delivered child number six. The other possibility could be another man in her life, which I did not want to discover, so I pulled his records to see if the six-week sperm count was negative.

"Congratulations on your new daughter. This is a surprise for both of us," I began over the telephone.

"Yes, it is, but we're both quite happy. I do think we should look into another vasectomy, however. That is much easier than having my tubes tied."

"Absolutely. Did your husband ever come in for the sperm count last year after his procedure? I don't see one in his records."

"No, he did not. I know that because I asked him to do it about a hundred times."

"OK. I'll get him to give me a sample soon, and obviously, that will show active sperm." I paused for a response. "There are not any other men in your life are there?"

"Doc, seriously? I had five children and a husband to take care of. No time in my life for another man," she laughed.

"Sorry. It's just a doctor-question I needed to ask before I get him back on the surgery table," I finish apologetically. "You know he is my first ever vasectomy failure."

I have made lots of mistakes over the years. I have given an elderly patient an antibiotic that caused kidney failure, and another patient took my prescribed medicines that resulted in heart failure.

I have missed lots of correct diagnoses that should not have been missed. I try to remember the long list of diagnostic guesses that have been proven incorrect because I learn much more from my patients than I do from medical books.

And I try very hard not to make the same mistake twice.

Chapter 70 – Sex

The topic of sex is often the last part of an office visit. Erectile dysfunction in men is common and treatable. Viagra is talked about and joked about in bars and locker rooms. For women, it is more commonly whispered between close friends, but if a doctor does not bring it up, sexual disorders are often missed.

"Mr. Ellington is here for his diabetes check. He says there's something else he wants to ask you, but he won't tell me what it is," began my medical assistant after completing the electronic medical check-in.

"Hey, Mr. Ellington, your sugars look better today. And the nurse says you have a question. Is it about a need for Viagra?" I smile. It usually is, and he nods.

A proper patient analysis includes a look at the many medicines that affect erections, life stressors, prostate and urination issues, smoking, and alcohol. The physical exam process provides the opportunity to discuss sexual matters each time a physical is done. For men, there is a brief pause while I pull on blue rubber gloves.

"OK, here comes the rubber-glove part of your exam. Please drop your trousers and underwear and face me. I need to check you for hernia and your testicles for lumps. Before we begin though, are you having a good urine stream?"

"Yes, Doc, no issues there, and I only get up once a night to pee, if that."

"Good, what about erections? Is that working, OK?" I always slip into the conversation.

"No. Glad you asked, actually. My wife wants me to try some Viagra," he uttered softly.

Prescription medicines are helpful, and there are some effective herbal preparations. Medications are frequently a source of dysfunction for men and women. Vaginal dryness, lack of interest in sex for men and women (libido), erection difficulties, premature and prolonged time to ejaculation, and sensitivity issues are common. If you don't ask, you won't find out about these problems that can destroy relationships.

Doctors are voyeurs into their patient's lives. The private revelations are often surprising.

"I want to have sex every night, but my husband is older, and he isn't very interested," volunteers my patient as we prepare for the pap smear. "He lets me go out to local bars periodically," she states.

"I see. Do you always use condoms? Have you had any issues with vaginal discharges?" I respond, trying to hide my surprise.

"I always use condoms. I keep them in my purse. And no issues with discharges."

"To be safe, why don't I do a swab for chlamydia and gonorrhea while we're doing your pap smear?" I add.

"OK, sure. Better to be safe than sorry," she shrugs. Alexia hands me the speculum, lubrication, and swab. She reaches in the drawer and adds a test tube that the STD swab will go into.

I paused to remember my residency rotation in adolescent medicine. It had turned out to be one long progression of teenaged men and women with sexually transmitted diseases. The patients presented one-after-another with green frothy vaginal discharges from chlamydia, milky fishy-smelling discharges from bacterial vaginosis, and warts surrounding the anus and vaginal lips and male foreskins. Sometimes the odor was overwhelming. I could not comfortably consider sex with my wife for a month until those visions dissipated.

Later that afternoon, a thirty-six-year-old lady came in with a new vaginal discharge. This is a common female complaint. Yeast infections after antibiotics, lubricated condoms with spermicides that irritate, and various sex lubricants can all lead to a vaginal odor or discharge.

She was a mother of two young teenagers, had discrete tattoos, and was a non-smoker. I started with the standard panel of questions looking for a reason for the discharge.

"Have you had any antibiotics lately or any menstrual issues?"

"No antibiotics, and my periods are regular."

"Any new sexual contacts?" I ask in a conversational tone.

"Well, yes. I went to a sex club in Arizona last week."

That caught me by surprise, so I took a moment to formulate my response. "Hmmm, was there more than one contact? Did you use condoms?"

"Yes. And no. It was a pretty wild time."

"OK, then to be safe, we should do tests for the most common sexually transmitted infections. This will include vaginal swabs and some blood tests for syphilis, hepatitis, and AIDS. Let me give you antibiotics today rather than wait for the results and cultures. OK?"

She nodded and looked relieved. When I read about sex clubs in Arizona that evening, I was reminded to ask later if she had sex with dogs or horses also, but had difficulty deciding how to work that into a future visit conversation.

I did ask later, and she denied it. But, one lesson taught early in school was that *everyone lies about sex.* The cultures came back negative for the common STD infections which I had treated her for. We continued her annual wellness exams and one more annual HIV lab to ensure the absence of infection. We did not need to speak of the past issues again to our mutual reliefs.

Certain strokes of the brain can destroy learned inhibitions that prevent usually suppressed thoughts and behaviors.

"Doctor, the eighty-year-old patient in room three needs you," began the giggling nurse. I was doing morning rounds on the inpatient hospital ward.

"OK. What's the problem?"

Giggling began again as two nurses came closer. "She has put the glass salt and pepper shakers into her vagina again. She did that last night too, and we found other items from her dinner tray were missing. We should warn you that she has had a stroke and is talking about sex in the most graphic terms, especially if a man comes in the room."

We all went in together, and they were correct that her graphic descriptions of what she wanted me to do to her made everyone blush, except her.

Homosexuality, transgender, and LGBTQ medical issues are hush-hush in public but need to be addressed in the doctor's office. Breast implants in men, sex reassignment surgery, female and male genital piercings, and external vaginal and anal warts needing treatment present with surprising frequency.

Sexually transmitted diseases are common, increasing in frequency, and keep local health departments busy. Child trafficking for sex is now an international epidemic. Medical journals have articles reminding providers to screen for human trafficking when a patient presents with unusual sexual histories. This underground crime network has been a source of wonder and distress over the years.

Chapter 71 – Medications

My approach to any new patient is to start with a review of their medications.

"OK, Janet, let's go through your list of medicines and see what we can get rid of," I start, and continue with the medications and vitamins that are the most concerning.

"Glucosamine/Chondroitin. Why are you taking that?" I ask.

"I think it's for my arthritis. My husband takes it," she answers.

"OK. Let's stop that one. It just causes expensive urine," I say smiling.

"The vitamin C causes kidney stones at the dose you're taking so stop that for now please. Your calcium is the wrong type and can clog your heart arteries. I like the vitamin D3, and since you take that, we can stop the calcium, " I counsel.

"We have learned over the years that the reason we advised women to take calcium was because doctors had not yet learned enough about vitamin D deficiency. It was the lack of vitamin D that was causing the low calcium. Let's keep going. At least I'm going to save you some money today," I recite again.

Patients appreciate being permitted to stop taking medicines that cost money and worry them about possible harm.

Pharmaceutical companies sell billions of dollars' worth of cholesterol-lowering drugs annually. Millions of patients have taken these medicines, but there is a high incidence of stopping them due to side effects.

They lower measurable lipid lab values but can cause liver toxicity, muscle pain, tendon rupture, kidney failure, anemia, joint pains, fatigue, and memory impairment, to name a few common issues seen. They raise blood sugars, lower testosterone levels in men and women, and can cause diabetes.

I have found it fascinating to watch my colleagues 'learn' about these drugs. We are bombarded with advertisements, and professional lectures. Pharmaceutical sales reps tout the difficult to believe benefits of various lipid medications. Cardiologists are heavily marketed, and as a result almost all compassionately believe that cholesterol medications are best given often and in the highest doses tolerated.

It is brilliant marketing. If the cardiologist insists on giving a patient any drug, it would be a brave primary care doctor that would argue against that plan. Fortunately, for some of my patients, I have learned to debate certain perceived benefits.

"Sir, the cardiologist I sent you to wants me to add a high-dose cholesterol-lowering drug to the medications you're currently taking. He wants me to add it because you have diabetes and a family history of heart trouble," I began.

"You're seventy-one years old and are on four medications for diabetes and hypertension. I need your input in deciding what we will do. There are currently no well-documented benefits from this medicine for anyone over the age of seventy-three. It costs you another co-pay each month. Side effects sometimes include higher sugars, fatigue, joint and muscle pains, liver and kidney issues, and memory problems," I stated.

"There's a statistically small possibility that the pill might prevent a future heart attack or a stroke, and the medical literature notes that it can reduce *non-fatal* cardiac events by thirty percent. But it has no known ability to help you live one month longer. What would you like to do, sir?"

"Doc, really? I already have memory issues, and my sugars are not doing that well. I'm not a rich man, and when I hit the insurance 'donut hole' in August, I'm not going to be able to afford the medicines I take now. You need to tell me what to do," he pleaded.

In my younger years as a physician, I believed what my teachers taught me, and prided myself on passing certification tests that routinely reminded me to give statins (a cholesterol drug) to my patients according to accepted lipid level guidelines. I memorized those guidelines, but those guidelines kept changing.

I received letters from local pharmacies asking me to give all my diabetic patients a statin drug, and even asking me to give my patients higher doses than the dose they saw I was already giving them. I find that insulting and disturbing. The sellers of these drugs are spending time and money telling doctors how they should practice. *How could that be permitted and accepted?* The answer is money.

"If it were me, I would not add this drug to the mix you're taking already. But, if you're worried about heart attacks or strokes, there might be a small benefit. It's difficult and expensive to find out if you might benefit. Technology is being developed to use genetics to test whether it could be useful, but that isn't ready yet. We could try a low dose to see how it affects you if you want to try it," I finish logically.

"No, thank you, Doc. I don't want more problems than I already have. I've already outlived my dad's age at his death and lost most of my friends. If there are any other meds you don't think I need, please get rid of those too," he pleaded.

We agreed to take a deep breath and wait.

"I'm OK with not using this now, but if you show any signs of heart trouble, I will want to start it. If you have a stroke or mini-stroke, we'll consider adding it. OK?" I conclude.

As he leaves, confused but trusting in my well-intentioned advice, I remember that my employer will continue to list me with a failing grade in the quality measures they use. They will not pay me the quality bonus I would earn if I gave more of these drugs to my patients. *Yes -- we were getting paid extra to prescribe these medicines.*

When I questioned the policy, I learned that a committee of well-intentioned doctors listed the prescribing of this drug as one of the quality-care measures for which our providers could earn extra money. I asked where the list of quality measures came from and discovered the list came from a medical insurance company.

How did insurance companies conclude that doctors giving statins to their insured patients represented quality care?

It is a good question. *Do the statin makers-and-sellers market the insurance agencies as hard as they market to doctors? Do they offer cost discounts for adding this to the quality lists?*

Will our patients forgive us for harming them in good faith? I hope so.

I push pills for a living and pray that I do some good. I like to tell folks that I have a pill for just about everything, but all drugs have side effects. A baby aspirin kills someone every day from uncontrollable bleeding. Tylenol is an effective suicide drug because the damage it causes to the liver is often irreversible and fatal. Diuretic 'water' pills can cause kidney failure.

Without a computer, it is dangerous to practice modern medicine. The interactions of different drugs are so frequent that only a computer can keep track. Pharmacies check for interactions, and electronic medical records give warnings when allergies or other issues are detected.

Our germs are becoming resistant to commonly used antibiotics, and allergic reactions to most antibiotics are common. These bacteria and viruses kill, and they are becoming harder to beat. The CDC notes that between 12,000 and 56,000 Americans die every year from the many types of flu viruses. The COVID-19 virus in 2020 killed even more. Without immunizations these numbers would be much higher.

In 1918, before the flu shot, the H1N1 flu virus infected one-third of the world's population and killed an estimated fifty-million people of all ages. The H1N1 virus is still out there but the typical flu shot protects against this and three other potentially fatal strains.

Immunizations and antibiotics have saved millions of lives and extended life expectancy worldwide. Horrible, potentially fatal diseases like smallpox have been wiped off the face of the earth. Urinary infections of the past were often fatal due to the lack of effective medications in everyday use today.

Over the years, my cardiology friends have sometimes added an observation when seeing my patients, "Doctor Adams may not agree with my statin recommendation, so I will leave that up to you and him."

They have learned over time, as I have, that diet, exercise, and lifestyle work better than any pill. The last five cardiac-disease patients of mine that died were all taking a statin and a baby aspirin. They all died before the age of sixty-six, at or before an age I had predicted. Cigarettes and lifestyle killed them, not cholesterol.

"Smoking will kill you," began my standard caring-toned lecture. But," I add, "if you quit now, the clock stops ticking." I look for a response.

"How will it happen?"
"I don't know. Lung cancer, bladder cancer, throat cancer, colon cancer, heart attack or stroke," I recite.

"Stroke is the worst, you know. You're not dead. Someone has to push you around in a wheelchair and feed and change you, but I'll be here when it happens and will help where I can. The clock is ticking loudly now, and if you want to quit, I can help."

I have noticed that this population of smokers lives a different life than most. They smoke and drink and experiment with drugs. They ride fast motorcycles and take chances. They tend to be more sexually promiscuous. They likely have more fun than I do, but they will deny their children and grandchildren their company much too early.

Chapter 72 – Military vs. Civilian

While in the Army, I worked in local hospitals doing inpatient and critical care on weekends. I met patients in the emergency room, admitted them to the hospital and intensive care wards, and managed them overnight.

There are several differences in how the civilian and military medical worlds operate. Many of these differences revolve around defensive medicine practiced to avoid malpractice lawsuits.

Out of uniform, I could no longer deliver my patients' babies. My malpractice insurance premiums would go up by $90,000/year if I delivered babies as I had done for years. In the military, the U.S. government insured us, so I enjoyed the opportunity to deliver my patient's children and watch them grow up.

> "The children
> oh, the children
> that I will have watched grow
> and healed and nourished
> and learned of life from
> and their world will be a tad better
> and mine great."
> Lisa Miller, MD, pediatrician

As civilian physicians, we order X-rays, lab tests, and consults to document what we already know. We spend the patients' and their insurance companies' money as fast as we can. Time is money and seeing as many patients as possible is how money is made in the insurance-fueled productivity-oriented medical world.

Military physicians attend teaching lectures, scrub in on surgeries, go to the field on exercises, provide emergency care on the ground after jumping out of airplanes, and go for a run to stay in shape. Military doctors need to pass the required annual physical fitness tests too.

There is no time in the fee-for-service world for non-revenue generating activities. This makes it hard to *walk the walk* we recommend to our patients to exercise daily, sleep, and eat well.

The military system worked well in primary care, but for surgical specialties, it was more difficult. Those specialists needed operating room experience. Time spent deployed, or in military training decreased the time doing what they needed to do – operate.

The military is changing how their hospitals and clinics are staffed. Congress has mandated that the military decrease the number of uniformed providers and staff. Civilian providers and staff will soon replace uniformed personnel. Leaders of hospitals and clinics may become contract employees. The current uniformed military medical system will be challenged. Which doctors will go to war with the soldiers is currently an unanswered question.

Medicines are generally cost-free to military families. Hospitalization does not bankrupt them, and emergency rooms are busy but well-staffed. Patients, including expectant mothers, infants, and the elderly, are usually seen and treated without billing hassles.

I miss that.

"It matters not how straight the gate,
How charged with punishments the scroll,
I am the master of my fate,
I am the captain of my soul."

Invictus – William Henley

Epilogue - First Do No Harm

"Doctor Adams, when you're finished with this patient, people from Human Resources want to speak with you. It looks like your last two patients are being moved to another provider," stated Alexia with confusion in her voice.

I knew what was going to happen next. I was going to lose my job.

I paused to think back on the many enjoyable years caring for patients in this town. We had moved here after the Army where I was welcomed as the town's first full-service family physician. The practice had exploded with patients and began winning Best Medical Office awards. So, I went to our local bank and pledged everything I owned -- or would ever earn - as collateral for a loan. Then with some physician partners, we built a new 14,000 square foot medical building on the main road through town.

Private practice had then become increasingly impractical due to cuts in private practice physician insurance payments. Large group practices did not see payment cuts. The 1945 McCarran-Ferguson Act had exempted insurers from federal antitrust oversight. They could price fix and share pricing information. Medical insurance companies were exempted from the anti-monopoly laws, so I had happily sold my practice to a hospital group for one dollar and signed on as an employee. That decision was going to bite me today.

I recalled asking a large insurer, at a medical conference, why they were price-fixing and pushing out the independent doctors, the response caused an audible gasp.

"We are a monopoly."

Medical systems management has lost touch with the most valuable resource in their organizations – providers like me. Doctors, nurse practitioners, and physician assistants generate one hundred percent of the income that pays their salaries, I recalled.

"You are being placed on administrative leave effective immediately while we investigate a reported statement you made," began the management physician tasked with delivering this news. He did not appear happy about it.

This meeting with corporate HR was not unexpected. I had dealt with support staff using the human resources system to protect themselves by filing trivial complaints before. In each past case, the complaining employees has lost their jobs, but I was held responsible and disciplined.

"Doc, please tell me you're not going to retire before I see you again," had asked many of my patients this last year.

"I promise you that I won't retire until coming to work stops being fun," I would always respond.

I am trained in fatal hand-to-hand combat techniques, lethal use of sticks, knives, and guns, and have maintained a fitness and weapons expertise that makes me a very unwelcome enemy. But the first two laws of combat if a fight is coming are, 1. *walk away,* and 2. *walk away.* If walking away is not possible, then the rule is – *there are no rules!*

"Even in a hero's heart, discretion is the better part of valor," (The Ghost, 1762), so I discussed the situation with my wife, shed a few tears, and contacted our CEO, a friend, to ask his permission to retire. He granted my request without question -- so I *walked away.*

The cost to replace a physician is estimated to be $100,000 to $500,000. Our clinic had been actively searching for another qualified MD for over a year with no success. My wife and family welcomed my retirement. It was mourned but accepted as well-earned by my patients.

I enjoy driving by the five-million-dollar multi-specialty medical building that we designed and built with my cardiology and surgery partners. It stands as a shining monument to our calculated risk-taking and eventual success.

I run into my past patients frequently, and they hug me, pray for me, and wish me well. I anticipate significant changes in our future medical care systems. It is inevitable.

Primum non nocere
First, do no harm.

CPSIA information can be obtained
at www.ICGtesting.com
Printed in the USA
LVHW052117220723
753132LV00010B/795